ST. ELIZABETH HOSPITAL MEDICAL CENTER
LIBRARY

D0077786

)1-1790

Psychiatric Differential Diagnosis

WILLIAM F. MAAG LIBRARY
YOUNGSTOWN STATE UNIVERSITY

WILLIAM F. MAAG LIBRARY
YOUNGSTOWN STATE UNIVERSITY

ST. ELIZABETH HOSPITAL MEDICAL CENTER *199*
SCHOOL OF NURSING LIBRARY.
1044 BELMONT AVE.
YOUNGSTOWN, OHIO 44501-1790

Psychiatric Differential Diagnosis

WITHDRAWN

Jeremy M. Pfeffer

BSc MB BS MRCP MRCPsych
Consultant Psychiatrist
Department of Psychiatry
The London Hospital
Whitechapel
London

Gillian Waldron

MB ChB MRCPsych
Consultant Psychiatrist
Department of Psychiatry
The London Hospital
Whitechapel
London

With contributions from

Dr J.C. Cookson

BM DPhil MRCP MRCPsych

Consultant Psychiatrist
The London Hospital
and
Deputy Director of the Joint Academic Unit of Human
Psychopharmacology of the London and St Bartholomew's
Hospital Medical Colleges

CHURCHILL LIVINGSTONE
EDINBURGH LONDON MELBOURNE AND NEW YORK 1987

40.00

CHURCHILL LIVINGSTONE
Medical Division of Longman Group UK Limited

Distributed in the United States of America by
Churchill Livingstone Inc., 1560 Broadway, New York,
N.Y. 10036, and by associated companies, branches
and representatives throughout the world.

© J Pfeffer and G Waldron 1987

All rights reserved. No part of this publication may be
reproduced, stored in a retrieval system, or transmitted in
any form or by any means, electronic, mechanical,
photocopying, recording or otherwise, without the prior
permission of the publishers (Churchill Livingstone, Robert
Stevenson House, 1–3 Baxter's Place, Leith Walk,
Edinburgh EH1 3AF).

First published 1987
Reprinted 1988

ISBN 0 443 03703 5

British Library Cataloguing in Publication Data
Pfeffer, Jeremy M.
    Psychiatric differential diagnosis.
    1. Mental illnesses — Diagnosis
    I. Title   II. Waldron, Gillian
    III. Cookson, J.C.
    618.89′075   RC469

Library of Congress-in Publication Data
Pfeffer, Jeremy M.
    Psychiatric differential diagnosis.

    1. Mental illness — Diagnosis. 2. Diagnosis,
Differential. 3. Psychiatry — Case studies. I. Waldron,
Gillian. II. Cookson, J.C. (John C.) III. Title.
[DNLM: 1. Diagnosis, Differential. 2. Mental Disorders —
diagnosis. WM 141 P524p]
RC473.D54P44   1987   616.89′075   86–26356

Printed and bound in Great Britain at The Bath Press, Avon

RC
473
.D54P44
1987

Preface

The vast majority of psychiatric text books are organized around diagnostic categories. However, patients present with symptoms and not diagnoses. In psychiatry many different distinct disorders may present with the same symptoms. It is on the further evaluation of these symptoms, by careful history taking and mental state examination, that the correct formulation can be made upon which to base a rational treatment plan. We therefore feel that the time is right for a book on psychiatry which approaches this field in the same way that patients do, i.e. via symptoms.

The format of the book is based on the highly successful *Tutorials in Differential Diagnosis*, each chapter dealing with different symptoms and ending with an illustrative case history. Secondly, we have chosen a variety of common presenting symptoms all of which may pose diagnostic difficulties both within psychiatric diagnoses and between psychiatric and physical ones.

This book is intended not only for trainee psychiatrists preparing for postgraduate examinations, principally Membership of the Royal College of Psychiatrists but also for medical students faced with psychiatry for the first time who may struggle to make sense of the lack of hard facts. It will also be useful for General Practitioners both in training and after qualification since the vast majority of psychiatric symptomatology is entirely managed in General Practice. It is hoped that it will be of use to general physicians whose patients frequently have psychiatric problems either exclusively or in addition to somatic pathology.

We are grateful to Dr John Cookson for his contributions to Chapters 3, 14, 16, and 17. We would also like to thank the publishers for permission to reproduce various items. Invaluable and patient help in the preparation of the manuscript was given by Theresa Clarke and Kim Hendrey. Last but not least we thank our spouses and families who tolerated our relative neglect of them and were unfailingly supportive and encouraging to us during the preparation of the book.

24298

WILLIAM F. MAAG LIBRARY
YOUNGSTOWN STATE UNIVERSITY

WILLIAM F. MAAG LIBRARY
YOUNGSTOWN STATE UNIVERSITY

Contents

1

The Assessment

The psychiatric process starts with the patient presenting (or being presented) with a problem to the therapist and ends with the successful resolution of that problem. The stages in between follow the same format as in any medical or scientific situation. This involves, firstly, ascertaining what the problem to be treated is, and secondly, formulating a working hypothesis upon which the third step, the treatment plan, can be based. In psychiatry the first part corresponds to the history, mental state, physical examination and further investigations, and the second step to the first part of the formulation which includes, but is not only, the diagnosis. The third step is self-evident, and is outside the remit of this book.

Table 1.1 The psychiatric history

Reason for Referral	
Complaints and history of present illness; presenting symptoms	Date of onset
	Precipitating factors
	Consistency
	Severity
	Exacerbating & relieving factors
	Nature
	Site & radiation
	Previous history of similar symptoms & treatment
	Family history of same
	Associated symptoms including change in sleep, appetite, weight & libido
Family history	Parents and siblings: dead or alive, ages, personality, occupation, marital stability
	Separation, bereavements
	Family psychiatric history
	Family medical history and current health
	Family relationships
Personal history	Childhood: birth, neurotic traits, behavioural problems, enuresis
	Adolescence
	Schooling and further education
	Occupation
	Psychosexual development
	Forensic
	Alcohol and drugs
	Past medical history
	Past psychiatric history
	Social circumstances
Personality	Premorbid and present if different
	Behaviour: actions and reactions
	Attitudes: self, others, sexual, authority
	Independence and responsibility
	Usual mood
	Religious beliefs, fantasy life
	Interests and hobbies

HISTORY

The patient should initially be allowed full rein to present his problem as he sees it. This should then be clarified by further prompting using open-ended questions or, if necessary, by direct closed-ended enquiry. At all times the interviewer must be empathic, receptive and non-judgmental. At the end of the interview he should summarize for the patient the salient points as he understands them and invite questions. This ensures that both doctor and patient are dealing with the same problem and shows the patient that the doctor is interested in him.

The following areas (see Table 1.1) must be covered by the history, which may take more than one interview. Understanding may be facilitated by use of visual aids such as life charts and family trees.

MENTAL STATE EXAMINATION

The mental state is the psychiatric equivalent of the physical examination and must be fully

Table 1.2 The mental state examination

Appearance and behaviour	Dress, facial expression, movement, behaviour on interview
Speech	Form and content Speed, flow, spontaneity, quantity, coherence Give verbatim examples
Mood	Subjective and objective Depression, anxiety, elation, anger, irritability, perplexity When abnormal particularize as with presenting symptoms (see Table 1.1)
Thought content	Preoccupations Morbid thoughts Obsessional ruminations and rituals
Abnormal beliefs	Ideas of reference Overvalued ideas Primary delusions: delusional ideas, mood and perception Delusions of persecutions; grandeur; poverty; self-deprecation; worthlessness; guilt; bodily ill-health; nihilism; love; infidelity and influence Other passivity phenomena including thought alienation: insertion, withdrawal and broadcast

Abnormal perception	Distortion: intensity, quality, form
	Illusion
	Hallucinations
	  Auditory: 2nd and 3rd person
	  Hearing one's thoughts spoken out loud
	  Visual
	  Olfactory
	  Gustatory
	  Tactile and somatic: includes passivity phenomena where the sensation is caused by others

Abnormal experiences of self and environment	Depersonalization Derealization Déja-vu Capgras syndrome
Cognitive state	Level of consciousness Orientation: time, place, person Attention and concentration Memory Intelligence
Insight	Appropriate awareness of illness Extent of understanding of causation
Rapport	

assessed and recorded on all occasions. It depends on accurate observations in addition to detailed questioning and follows a systematic format (see Table 1.2).

PHYSICAL EXAMINATION

Where indicated the patient should be physically examined.

FURTHER ASSESSMENT

Information gathering

The information base on which the formulation is made is increased by interviewing other informants, including the general practitioner, other involved care givers, spouse, family and friends and by reading medical notes. Continuing interviews with the patient, both alone and together with spouse and family, and further clarification of the mental state including, where relevant, a detailed assessment of higher cerebral function further increase the information available, as do social enquiry, nursing and occupational therapy assessment.

Investigations

These include the following:

Laboratory tests	— e.g. blood and urine tests, X-rays, EEG and CAT scan
Psychological testing	— for cognitive function including memory, intelligence and specific deficits and the more subjective personality and psychopathology assessments
Questionnaires	— for mental state, personality and life events
Behavioural analysis	— including sleep and behaviour charts

FORMULATION

The formulation is a concise and rational method of defining the problems presented by the patient which should lead logically through the process of symptoms, diagnosis and management. It is not only applicable to psychiatry but also to other branches of medicine and is a way of making an imprecise and potentially woolly topic into one where the scientific method can, at least to some extent, be applied.

There are many different ways of constructing a formulation. The following is one scheme and consists of five sections — introduction, diagnosis, aetiology, management and prognosis — which form a logical progression.

Introduction

The introduction should be a re-statement in about four sentences of the history, mentioning only relevant positive or negative points. The first sentence presents demographic data and the presenting problem in chronological order together with any precipitating events. An example of this would be: 'Mrs Jones is a 24-year-old married housewife and mother of three young children, who presents with a history of one year's headaches, six months' breathlessness and four weeks' inability to leave the house following the birth of her youngest child'.

The second sentence presents relevant information about the family history, and the third covers the personal history.

The fourth sentence concerns relevant features of the mental state including any difficulties in taking the history, and physical factors where appropriate.

Any of the topics covered in these four sentences may need to be very slightly elaborated so that the four sentences may turn into five, or at the most six; but it should never be more than a precis of the facts and should never be just a rehash of the history.

Taking our hypothetical Mrs Jones a stage further, the introductory paragraph may read as follows: 'Mrs Jones is a 24-year-old married housewife and mother of three young children who presents with a history of one year's headaches, six months' breathlessness and four weeks' inability to leave the house following the birth of her youngest child. Her parents were divorced when she was young and her mother has a history of anxiety. Her childhood was unsettled, there were episodes of school refusal; she married at the age of twenty and there have been communication and sexual difficulties in the marriage. She has always been anxious and somewhat houseproud and was given tranquillizers at the time of her marriage and the birth of her first two children. The mental state reveals an anxious and tearful lady who complains of a worried and unhappy mood with initial insomnia and psychic, somatic and phobic symptoms of anxiety; the physical examination was normal'.

Diagnosis

A diagnosis is a shorthand way of describing what is wrong with the patient. However, though this may be suitable in most medical circumstances there are problems in applying it to psychiatry. The diagnosis should provide therapeutic and prognostic indicators but in psychiatry these are often relatively weak. In addition the diagnosis may be inadequate to describe the patient's predicament and the majority of patients do not conform to stereotypes. Furthermore, there may be harmful effects from attaching a name to a condition and thus implying an understanding greater than that which actually exists. Too heavy an emphasis on diagnosis may lead to the treatment of diseases rather than people. Finally a diagnostic label, even if wrong, once attached is difficult to remove. Nevertheless a diagnosis is important for communication, research and epidemiology, but because of these shortcomings it is important that one produces a longer formulation.

There are two major international classificatory systems for diagnosis. The first is the International Classification of Diseases — ICD–9* (see Appendix I) — which classifies people on a single psychiatric axis, and is the system most commonly used in this country. The second is the Diagnostic and Statistical Manual — DSM-III (see Appendix II) — which is the system used in the U.S.A., which classifies people on five different axes: psychiatric illness, personality disorder, physical illness, severity of psychological stressors, and highest level of adaptive functioning. One of the main

* ICD–10 is under preparation at the time of writing

advantages of the DSM–III lies in its separation of personality disorders from psychiatric illness, as both may exist either separately or together. Even where no personality disorder *per se* exists a brief description of the premorbid personality is useful at this stage as it has major implications for the following sections. It is also important to mention here intelligence if relevant (usually where the patient is of low intelligence).

When discussing illness, a differential diagnosis should be presented explaining the reasons for each interpretation. The most likely should be first and only those which fit the facts should be included. There may be more than one psychiatric illness, for example depression and alcoholism, and physical illnesses may also be present. When only one diagnosis fits all the facts, no differential should be given.

Aetiology

The third section concerns the question, 'Why has *this* person presented at *this* time with *these* symptoms?'. This can be considered both in physical, dynamic, behavioural and sociocultural terms, and on a temporal basis with reference to long term, intermediate and precipitating factors. Long term is from conception to adulthood and includes adverse effects of genetic endowment, prenatal and birth trauma and childhood experiences. Intermediate factors concern personality difficulties, e.g. areas of ongoing vulnerability, and longstanding situational difficulties, life events and previous psychiatric history.

Management

Management can be divided into three parts: further assessment, and management of both the acute and long term conditions. As stated above, further assessment will increase the information on which the detailed treatment plan is based. The treatment of the acute illness should be considered on one or more of four lines-physical, dynamic, behavioural and social. (see Table 1.3). It is important to state how treatment and further assessment should be carried out: as an in-patient, out-patient or day-patient; voluntarily or under the Mental Health Act 1983; who should carry it out; for how long it should last and what the aim

Table 1.3 Methods of treatment

Physical	Drugs, ECT, psychosurgery
Psychotherapeutic	Supportive, counselling, interpretative Individual, group, marital, family
Behavioural	General, e.g. anxiety management Specific, e.g. social skills, sex therapy, cognitive therapy.
Social	Occupational, housing, social network and leisure

or desired outcome should be. Long term treatment can be considered along the same lines.

Prognosis

In each patient one should balance favourable and unfavourable prognostic factors. The prognosis

Table 1.4 Formulation

Introduction	1 Demographic data, symptoms, precipitating events	
	2 Family history	
	3 Personal history	
	4 Mental state and physical examination	
Diagnosis	1 Personality	
	2 Psychiatric illness	
	3 Physical illness	
Aetiology		
Cause	1 Physical	
	2 Dynamic	
	3 Behavioural	
	4 Sociocultural	
Time	1 Long term	Prebirth including Genetic Childhood
	2 Mid term	Personality difficulties Life events and ongoing situational difficulties Previous psychiatric history
	3 Short term	Immediate precipitants
Management	1 Further assessment	information gathering tests and observations
	2 Of acute disorder	physical psychotherapeutic behavioural socioenvironmental
	3 Long term	physical psychotherapeutic behavioural socioenvironmental
Prognosis	Illness itself	
	Modifying factors in patient, environment and treatment	
	1 Short term	
	2 Long term	

can be divided into short term and long term forecasts; these are not necessarily the same, in that while an acute illness may respond very favourably to treatment, the patient may be subject to recurrences at frequent intervals. The prognosis depends on the nature of the illness itself; for example, senile dementia (Alzheimer's disease) carries an intrinsically poorer prognosis than the potentially reversible dementia of myxoedema. However, the illness can only occur in the context of the patient and, therefore, the prognosis is dependent on the particular features of his illness, his previous history, his compliance and motivation, his response to treatment, his social support system and any prevailing stresses. Thirdly the prognosis depends on variables in the treatment, including availability, therapist competence and unwanted effects.

TO CONTINUE THE SAGA OF MRS JONES

Diagnosis

a) Premorbid personality
   Anankastic personality disorder (ICD 301.4)
   Psychosexual personality difficulties
b) Psychiatric differential diagnosis
   1 *Anxiety state* (300.0)
   2 *Phobic state (agoraphobia)* (300.2)
   3 *Neurotic depression* (300.4)
   4 *Adjustment reaction* (309.2)
   5 *Frigidity* (302.7)

The presenting symptoms of headache and breathlessness in the presence of a normal physical examination, and associated mood disturbance, suggest that these are somatic symptoms of anxiety. Despite the presence of phobic symptoms which might suggest a diagnosis of *agoraphobia* (300.2) this has arisen in the setting of many months' somatic and psychic symptoms of anxiety of a free-floating non-situational type which dominates the clinical picture and therefore leads to the diagnosis of *anxiety state* (300.0). Similarly although the presence of unhappiness is at first sight consistent with a diagnosis of *neurotic depression* (300.4), in this case the depression is secondary to the anxiety rather than being either primary or equal in importance to it. In addition though this illness has followed the stress of child-birth and might lead one to a diagnosis of *adjustment reaction* (309.2) the past history of a long relapsing course following various different stresses is probably more in keeping with the diagnosis of anxiety state.

As for the sexual dysfunction, if it had arisen only in the context of the disturbance of mood, it would not warrant a diagnostic label of its own. However further assessment shows that Mrs Jones has a long history of sexual problems such as avoidance of intercourse even at times when her mood has been stable. Hence the additional diagnosis of *frigidity* (302.7).

In summary therefore the diagnosis for psychiatric illness is:

1 Anxiety state   (300.0)
2 Frigidity   (302.7)

Aetiology

Models

a Physical
There may possibly be a genetic component in that the mother had a history of anxiety.

b Behavioural
Mother's history of agoraphobia may have been learned by the patient as a way of coping with problems. The same is likely to be true of the episodes of school refusal.

c Dynamic
The fact that her parents were divorced when she was young may have led both to insecurity and to psychosexual problems including ambivalence in accepting her role as a wife and mother. The former is borne out by the childhood history of school refusal and her anxious personality, and the latter by the sexual difficulties and the need for tranquillizers at the time of her marriage and the birth of her children.

d Sociocultural
She may have an inadequate social support system to help her physically and emotionally in the care of her three young children.

Her social isolation may have been further exacerbated by her agoraphobia.

Aetiology by time

Long term
Mother had agoraphobia
School refusal as a child
Parents' divorce

Mid term
a Personality difficulties:
her anxious and obsessional personality has made her likely to develop anxiety and depression under stress.
Her long history of psychosexual difficulties suggests that events associated with sexuality are particularly stressful.

b Life events and long standing situational difficulties:
The presence of post-puerperal anxiety states after her first two births may have led her to expect the same after this birth.
The long-standing marital problems have left her unsupported and may have led to an increased emotional investment in this child and/or to this pregnancy been unwanted.

c Past psychiatric history:
The past history of anxiety states after stress suggests a predisposition to a similar reaction in other stressful situations.

Immediate precipitants
The birth of her third child was the most likely precipitating event.
The somatic symptoms of anxiety may have set up a vicious circle.

Management

Further assessment
interview husband and mother
communicate with GP to obtain details of previous history
marital diagnostic interview
family interview

Investigations
A behavioural analysis might identify which activities or events lead to an increase or decrease in anxiety.

Treatment of Acute Illness

Where
Treatment should be home based or as an outpatient

By whom
Initially the general practitioner or a behaviour therapist, with the co-operation of the family. If there is no improvement a psychiatrist may become involved as may a psychotherapist.

How long
Problems needing relatively short-term treatment include the agoraphobia, the somatic and psychic symptoms of anxiety and possibly the marital and sexual situation although this may extend into the long term.

Treatment approaches
1 Physical:drugs:
  minor tranquillizers only to be used very short-term as an adjunct to behaviour therapy.
  sedative tricyclic antidepressants or monoamine oxidase inhibitors as a reserve line of treatment.

2 Psychotherapy:
  interpretative; individual or group, depending on intellect, verbal ability and availability of skilled therapist.
  support and counselling
  marital therapy which also includes a behavioural component.

3 Behavioural:
  relaxation and breathing training
  in vivo exposure/desensitization for agoraphobia.
  sex therapy

4 Socio-cultural:
  social contact with other mothers of young children
  increase personal outlets
  consideration of nursery placement for one or both of the elder children if appropriate to their needs.

Long term treatment
1 Physical:
  depends on remaining symptoms
2 Psychotherapy:
  interpretative or supportive
3 Behavioural:
  this should be short term
4 Social:
  increase social outlets

Prognosis

Short term
Good for agoraphobia and disturbance of mood
Less certain for marital, sexual and personality problems

Long term
The nature of phobic anxiety states is to run a relapsing course and in this woman one may expect further problems at times of psychosexual stress, e.g. further childbirth, menopause, children leaving home; and separations — loss of parents or spouse.

WILLIAM F. MAAG LIBRARY
YOUNGSTOWN STATE UNIVERSITY

2

Disorders of appearance

In the standard examination of the mental state 'appearance and behaviour' head the list, largely to underline the fact that significant clues to psychosocial function can be gathered before the patient speaks (see Table 1.2) and to stress that observation, an apparently simple technique, must not be overlooked in the desire to understand symptoms. This is a cardinal maxim of clinical examination throughout medicine and in this respect, psychiatry is not unusual.

Appearance can, for the purpose of this chapter, be usefully, if arbitrarily, divided into two parts: that over which one has no control, and that over which one exercises choice. Hence physical characteristics such as height, baldness, and noticeable birth marks are not a matter of personal choice and are either unchangeable or modifiable only with difficulty; whereas style of dress and personal possessions are, in an affluent society, a matter of individual choice. The way in which a person dresses states his sense of congruence with his social surroundings, but also may express the extent to which he values appearance, or his aspirations to be part of a particular subgroup of society. Many, perhaps most, cultures have more or less subtle, unwritten codes whereby one's position in the social hierarchy is betrayed by the adoption of different styles of dress, speech or nonverbal communication. (The role of uniform in this respect is revealing as an indicator of status, whether the wearer is in a leadership or subservient role, and at the same time is an indicator of social and personal equality with all others with the identical uniform.) This chapter concerns the psychiatric significance of aberrations of appearance. Some aspects of behaviour are so intricately interwoven with appearance that they will be touched on here, but extreme disturbances of behaviour are considered elsewhere.

Psychiatrists and others concerned with the mentally ill must be constantly alive to the need not to be arbiters of 'correct' social behaviour — not to judge eccentricity and individuality as illness merely because they take different or unpopular forms. Nowhere is this danger so marked as in the observation of people's appearance and care must be taken not to overinterpret the unusual. Looking odd is not the same as being odd — an eccentrically dressed individual is not necessarily mentally ill and neither is the cerebral palsied patient, although society all too often treats him as such. For diagnostic purposes the essential aspect of appearance is its congruence with the patient's life style; in other words, use the individual as his own control. For example, if a middle-aged successful businessman who has always been punctilious about his neat and sober clothing appears at work dressed in caftan and beads, then it would be reasonable to look for other features in his mental state suggesting mania. Alternatively, if over the space of weeks he becomes shabby, unkempt and dirty, then one should suspect marital break-up, alcoholism or an organic dementing process.

DISORDERS OF PHYSICAL APPEARANCE

Physical abnormalities may result from disease, be self-inflicted or exist only in the mind of the patient. We will consider these in turn.

WILLIAM F. MAAG LIBRARY
YOUNGSTOWN STATE UNIVERSITY

Physical appearance caused by disease

Congenital or acquired physical disability is accompanied by psychological difficulties which vary in intensity according to the patient's personality, mental state and past experiences, and his inter-relationships with other people. Thus the extent of loss of function and deprivation of activity, and the importance of damage in a particular site or to a particular organ, may vary from person to person. Psychiatric help may particularly be required at the recovery phase, when optimum function and adjustment to disability are not realised because of grieving, denial or depression. However, disfiguring conditions, whilst dependent for their impact on very much the same variables as disabling ones, have a different emphasis inasmuch as function is usually minimally impaired, but appearance substantially so. The extent to which society values appearance, the existence of superstitions about aberrant characteristics, and the sex role expectations within the culture are extrapersonal factors which modify adjustment. For example, women present with psychological problems about baldness or facial disfigurement more often than men.

Severe facial disfigurement, such as naevi, scars from accidents or burns, or cleft lip, may permanently impair appearance despite remedial surgery and recent advances in cosmetic camouflage. Psychiatric difficulties as a result are largely linked to social anxiety. Avoidance of other people is reinforced by the behaviour of others, whether it be a sympathetic avoidance of staring or a horrified or disgusted reaction. Perhaps because of this component of reality in the socially phobic disfigured patient, presentation to the psychiatrist is relatively uncommon and severely affected persons may become totally housebound and reclusive. Many such persons never expose themselves to sexual rejection and never form either superficial or intimate relationships. Appearance is highly symbolic and is often seen as a 'window' to the inner personality; hence disfigured patients may perceive themselves and be perceived as bad all through, and may be severely and chronically depressed.

Less severe or transient abnormalities may be revealed as problems in the course of the consultation. Skin rashes, especially acne in adolescents, contribute to anxiety about social and sexual success at a time when confidence is likely in any case to be low. Similar difficulties present in patients with disordered body size, for example dwarfism and obesity.

Patients who experience mutilating trauma or surgery have been the subject of many psychiatric studies, and long term psychiatric sequelae have been identified in between 25 and 60 per cent of most series. The type of disorder varies with the type of illness and its continuing threat to health or life, but some mutilations are seen to have particular significance. Mastectomy, for example, provokes major stress in women about their femininity and attractiveness, whilst colostomy is regarded by many as a horrifying problem in social situations. Anxiety, depression and sexual problems are particularly common in these patients.

Though disfigurement often leads to psychiatric problems a diagnostic pitfall is to assume that the psychiatric condition is entirely explained by the patient's disfigurement with a failure to notice the extent to which she or he hides other psychological problems behind it. For example, 'Everyone stares at me' may be true or it may mask an accompanying paranoid state.

Self-induced disorders of appearance

Self-mutilation

Repetitive self-inflicted injury, usually in the form of superficial cuts to hands, arms and face, is a feature of some patients with personality disorders. The resulting lesions are commonly not severely disfiguring although there is a wide variation in behaviour. The medial aspect of the forearm is a frequent site of parallel scars in such patients. They usually admit that these injuries are self-inflicted, although they may claim to have no memory of the event, which leads some to classify this as a dissociative response.

Dermatitis artefacta

Self-inflicted skin injury is classified as dermatitis artefacta in patients who present to dermatologists, usually deny that the lesions are self-inflicted, and produce lesions which are not at first sight obviously self-inflicted, for example, ones caused by knives, scissors and needles. Lesions in dermatitis artefacta are often large, superficially necrotic and have a clear geometric shape. They are slow to heal since the patient continues to damage the skin, but heal normally when covered by an occlusive bandage in hospital, where the patient is observed. Patients with dermatitis artefacta are usually young women, often in nursing or related professions, and may have a long history of investigation and treatment for physical complaints and evidence of personality disorder. They rarely admit that they harm themselves and this condition can be seen as part of the group of disorders, of which the Munchausen syndrome is the most spectacular, which are characterised by gross dependence on patient-hood, gratification from illness and the pain and discomfort of surgical and investigative procedures, primary or secondary narcotic dependence, little or no satisfying non-hospital life, rapid change of medical attendants and complete denial of and resistance to a psychiatric interpretation.

Perceived disorders of appearance

Dymorphophobia

Strictly speaking, dysmorphophobia is neither a phobia nor a disorder of appearance, but in practice there is no condition where appearance dominates the clinical interview as markedly as does this. A patient with dysmorphophobia believes that some part of his or her body is disfigured or misshapen. The most common parts of the body which are subject to this belief are those which are exposed, such as the face or ears, or associated with sexual attractiveness, such as the breasts. Objectively there is little or nothing abnormal in appearance. Characteristically the patient will fail to be reassured by the opinion of others as to the normality of the part in question, either believing that people are lying about their appearance, or, in those with more insight, stating that it is his or her own opinion that matters, not that of others.

Transient dysmorphophobic feelings may be a feature of adolescence or present in people with sensitive insecure personalities and low self-esteem. The persistent symptom is correctly classified as either an overvalued idea or a delusion. It is an overvalued idea when there is a degree of objective reality — for example, the patient's nose is slightly larger, or her breasts slightly smaller than average — but this then preoccupies the patient who attributes his or her difficulties disproportionately to it. Such a patient can manage to obtain a more normal perspective from time to time, but this seldom lasts long. Deluded patients, however, are totally convinced that they are disfigured, that this is the cause of all their difficulties; and are quite untouched by rational argument, or interpretations that they are expressing feelings about themselves and not solely their bodies.

Such patients usually request cosmetic surgery and may present to the psychiatrist via the plastic surgeon. Some patients present to the psychiatrist only after surgery has been carried out, when, not surprisingly, they feel that they look no better and request further surgery to correct the previous operation, although sometimes surgery may improve the symptoms. On rare occasions, patients may feel so desperate about their appearance that they attempt to precipitate plastic surgery by mutilating themselves, or request quite impossible corrective surgery, to lengthen their penis or totally to alter their face.

Severe dysmorphophobia totally disrupts the patient's life in that he becomes socially phobic and will not expose himself to the view of others more than he can help, and dysmorphophobia occasionally underlies a presentation of agoraphobia. Although dysmorphophobia alone is not a symptom of depressive illness, secondary depression is sometimes present and exacerbates the clinical picture.

Delusional dysmorphophobia is classified as a monosymptomatic delusional psychosis, but is usually associated with symptoms of severe personality problems in other respects. It may also be a symptom of acute schizophrenia, and here other schizophrenic symtoms will be present (see chapter 17) and the complaint of abnormality may be exceptionally bizarre.

Studies of the natural history of the condition indicate that a significant minority develops schizophrenia in later years, and that it remains in most patients a chronic disabling condition, difficult to alleviate.

INAPPROPRIATE CONCERN ABOUT PHYSICAL APPEARANCE

Many people resent the passage of years and the commensurate decline in their appearance, strength and agility. Old age is highly associated with psychiatric illness, but anxiety about the consequences of ageing may present in young adult patients where the change of appearance and reduction of sexual attractiveness are most feared. It is most commonly found in narcissistic egocentric personalities who always take great care with their appearance, clearly give a high priority to fashion and glamour and are usually flirtatious. Their social and sexual relationships are characterized by instant success, on first impressions, followed by failure to maintain the relationship once the first excitement has passed. As the years go by, the realization that the attractive power is beginning to wane often produces a desperate desire to remain young, with increasingly inappropriate grooming and dress, before the reality becomes inescapable and the patient may become markedly depressed. The patient's poor sense of self-worth is usually easy to elicit, together with an awareness that he or she relies on outside appearance for want of anything else to offer. Undue dependence on the external trappings of clothes, possessions and status should be identified if present in any consultation since it is indicative that self-esteem is preserved in this way rather than experienced inside the self and heralds difficulties when or if the shell cannot be maintained.

LACK OF SELF CARE

The opposite end of the spectrum from extreme concern with personal appearance is total disregard for it, and although it must be remembered that there is a wide variation in normal interest in and priority given to external appearance, changes in self-care are important clinical signs in psychiatry. Acute deterioration in standards of dress, cleanliness and household tasks may be a prominent, indeed the presenting sign of a serious depressive illness. Organic brain disease is also a cause, because of disinhibition and a change of self-awareness, as a result of dressing apraxia in parietal lobe lesions or because of generalized disorientation and memory loss. Acute schizophrenia can result in acute self-neglect because of specific delusions such as a fear of washing because of poisoned water in the bathroom; or because the patient is too preoccupied by his experiences to pay attention to everyday living. Similarly, manic patients may be too busy with exciting schemes to care to change their clothes, or they may adopt uncharacteristic, usually highly colourful, styles of dress.

Chronic self-neglect is a prominent feature of chronic schizophrenia, where drive and motivation to maintain daily activities are impaired. Alcohol and drug dependence, and dementia, are also important causes.

Poor standards of family and domestic hygiene may be present in the absence of definable psychiatric illness. Chaotic families characterized by repeated marital break-up, violence, alcohol abuse, debt, delinquency, eviction, truancy of children and either insufficient or inappropriate and excessive use of Health and Social Services often have a very poor standard of self-care and hygiene for their families. Wives and mothers in these families have often grown up in similar households and may have had little or no opportunity to learn appropriate skills. They may be of low intelligence, and poverty, although not an invariable accompaniment, obviously exacerbates the situation. Depression, common in mothers with young families, is a diagnosis to be considered and is likely if there has been a clear, recent change in their coping ability. However, although intermittent depression of mood is an almost invariable accompaniment of such a lifestyle, signs of depressive illness as such are usually lacking in families with a chronic inability to cope domestically.

A similarly poor level of domestic care has been described in some elderly patients in the absence of psychiatric illness, and called the senile squalor syndrome. This may be associated with apathy and a sense of alienation in the elderly patient who may have had a precarious ability to care for himself or herself in the past. Most cases of squalid domestic circumstances in the elderly, however, are attributable to gross physical incapacity and/or dementia or depressive illness.

Table 2.1 Psychiatric illnesses reflected in appearance

Feature	Variation	Indicates
Level of consciousness	Drowsy, clouded	Acute confusional state
	Sudden onset of sleep out of clear consciousness	Narcolepsy
Gait	Exaggerated abnormality	Attention-seeking personality
	Shuffling	Idiopathic/drug induced parkinsonism
	Weakness	Neurological disorder (?? hysteria)
	Ataxia	Alcohol or drug intoxication, neurological disorder, hysteria
Self care 1 dress	a Sexually inappropriate	Sexual identity difficulties
	b Inappropriate for age and class	Personality difficulties Depression Mania Schizophrenia
2 personal hygiene	Poor	Alcohol/drug addiction Depression Chronic schizophrenia Dementia
Facial expression 1 constant	Impoverished, absent expression	Depression, Parkinson's disease
	Mouth & eye corners turned down Vertical furrows in forehead	Depression
	Tears in eyes or falling	Grief, sadness
	Eyes wide open, pupils dilated	Anxiety
	Horizontal furrows in forehead	Anxiety
	Eye contact avoided	Anxiety; suspicion
	Prolonged eye contact; clenched teeth	Hostility
2 intermittent	Eyes & head gazing around	Distractability confusional state hypomania, paranoid psychosis
	Eyes diverting away to one point with expression of concentration	Auditory hallucinations
Facial features	Absence of hair and eyebrows	Alopecia Hair pulling
	Heavy overgrowth of jaw, supraorbital structures	Acromegaly
suggesting mental impairment	Small head, receding chin and forehead	Microcephaly
	Gross enlargement of skull	Hydrocephalus
	Epicanthic fold, Brushfields spots on iris, small nasal bridge, short thick neck, hypertelorism, ptosis	Down's syndrome Other trisomies
	Adenoma sebaceum	Tuberose sclerosis
	Port wine stain on half face	Sturge-Weber syndrome
	Large head, frontal bossing, low set ears	Hurler's syndrome

Table 2.1 (*cont'd*)

Feature	Variation	Indicates
Posture	Sits forward on edge of chair	Anxiety
	Slumped, hunched body	Depression
	Tense, clenched fists	Anger
	Inappropriately relaxed e.g. lies back, feet on desk	Hypomania
Hands and arms (*see chapter on movement*)	Pill rolling tremor	Parkinson's disease Extrapyramidal syndrome
	Trembling & sweaty palms	Anxiety state
	Excoriation of hands	Obsessional hand-washing
	Scars of self-inflicted wounds	Deliberate self-harm

CASE HISTORY

ANGELA MILLER

Angela, a 21-year-old single girl, was referred for a psychiatric opinion by her GP. She attended reluctantly, stating that her only reason for coming was so that she could obtain a psychiatric recommendation for cosmetic surgery on the NHS — on the grounds that failure to have surgery was causing her psychological distress.

About a year ago, Angela had given up her undergraduate course in history because she was increasingly unable to attend lectures because of anxiety. She had progressively given up all social activity and was now virtually housebound, apart from a weekly visit to sign on as unemployed and local shopping for essential foods. She avoided all activity which brought her into contact with others because she could not bear people looking at her. The only person she talked to was her boyfriend with whom she had lived for eighteen months. They planned to get married in six months' time and Angela was already stating that he could meet and mix with other people on their honeymoon but she would stay in their room. She totally denied that any of this was a problem, saying that she was quite happy on her own, that she had no ambitions for career or a social life, and that her behaviour was not abnormal.

Three years before, Angela had had cosmetic surgery to reduce the prominence of her ears. Six months before referral she had expensive private cosmetic surgery on both breasts to reduce their size but she was dissatisfied with the result. She and her boyfriend had borrowed a large amount of money to pay for this. She now requested further surgery; to correct the previous unsatisfactory breast operations and to alter the shape and appearance of her face. Although she could not afford this she said she was prepared somehow to find the money if necessary.

There was no family history of psychiatric trouble. She was an only child, born to an older couple who were remote and cold in their relationship. She remembered little emotional warmth in the home and recalled her father using violence to her mother on several occasions. She was clever at school and encouraged to achieve academically at the expense of social relationships; her parents did not encourage her to develop friendships or to go out with boys. Her current boyfriend was her first, and she had had no previous sexual experience.

She had unexpectedly failed her A-level examinations three years ago, and re-sat them a year later after leaving school and studying at home. She left home for the first time to attend university, which she initially enjoyed, sharing a flat with other girls.

The relevant features of the mental state examination were that her appearance was of an exceptionally pretty girl who was excessively and grossly made-up, who avoided eye contact and whose mood was either anxious and hesitant or sullen and defiant. She denied any psychiatric problems and said that her need for surgery was so self-evident that a search for such problems was not only unnecessary but an insult to her intelligence. She said that the opinion of her mother and boyfriend, that her appearance did not need changing, was irrelevant.

Questions

What is the likely differential diagnosis?
What important aetiological factors are present?
Why does this problem present now?
What advice should be given on further surgery?

The initial diagnosis of dysmorphophobia is obvious. Angela's only complaints over the last three years have been of dissatisfaction with the shape of her ears, her breasts, and her whole face. Although the objective evidence about the initial appearance of her ears and breasts cannot now be commented on, there is no apparent abnormality of her face. The total conviction of her belief coupled with requests for surgery which are increasing in frequency indicates that her dysmorphophobic beliefs are held with delusional intensity. Although there is no other evidence of psychotic thinking or experience, the natural history of the condition would indicate that the future development of schizophrenia is a risk. At present the diagnosis is of monosymptomatic delusional psychosis — of dysmorphophobia. Her avoidance of social situations indicates a social phobia secondary to the dysmorphophobia but she is not complaining of this.

The aetiology is unclear but long term environmental factors suggest themselves, centering perhaps on her experience as a loveless, rejected child, born (unexpectedly and unwillingly?) to parents who did not express affection. Her self-concept of an unlovable child may have been fixed on to a belief that her appearance was unlovable but this requires further elucidation. Medium term factors may have been her academic failure (affecting the only aspect of her that her parents valued), which preceded her first surgery; and the recent triggers her failure at university and her impending marriage, which poses a threat because of her undeveloped sexuality.

The problem presents now principally because she has no money. If she had been able to afford to have further surgery privately she would not have seen a psychiatrist at all. Care must be taken not to overinterpret the significance of presentation to a psychiatrist in such a case, but it must also be acknowledged that the fact that Angela knew she would be refused surgery on the NHS (in the absence of psychiatric approval), indicates some insight; and her presentation now might indicate awareness of the likelihood of future difficulties upon marriage.

Further surgery would be disastrous. The evidence that many people who seek cosmetic surgery are improved psychologically as a result is irrelevant to this case. Despite two operations she remains totally dissatisfied with her appearance and is asking for increasingly unrealistic procedures.

Funny movements

Although abnormal movements might seem at first to be the province of the neurologist rather than the psychiatrist, they do in practice have important associations with psychiatry. Firstly the motor manifestations may be the most prominent symptoms of certain psychiatric disorders, for instance the immobility of the stuporose patient, the manifestations of catatonia and the variety of hysterical conversion symptoms. Secondly neuropsychiatric disorders (e.g. Huntington's Chorea, Parkinson's disease) involve both extrapyramidal neurological signs and psychological symptoms. Thirdly drugs administered by psychiatrists may have side-effects evoking abnormal movements and it may be difficult to assess the significance of these in the overall clinical picture. Fourthly, purely neurological disorders affecting, for instance, the movements of expression may be

misinterpreted in psychological terms (e.g. hemifacial spasm).

The most valuable aid to diagnosing abnormal movements is previously to have seen and recognized the condition in question. The diagnosis may immediately be obvious in which case attention will soon turn to elucidating the aetiology (e.g. of Parkinsonism), but further examination and assessment may be needed. The different neurological disorders are defined in Table 3.1.

TREMOR

Tremors can be further defined according to whether they occur in a part of the body that is relaxed and supported (resting or static tremor), when the part is held in a posture (postural tremor), or when the part is deliberately moving (action tremor or intention tremor). The frequency of oscillation of the tremor is also of diagnostic importance. The lowest frequency is the postural tremor associated with multiple sclerosis (2–3 c/s); the Parkinsonian resting tremor including pill-rolling of the hand occurs slightly faster at 4–5 c/s. A postural tremor at 6 c/s may occur in tired limbs after exertion or may be an 'essential tremor' with autosomal dominant inheritance. A higher frequency of postural tremor (6.5–11 c/s) is the 'physiological tremor' which may become exaggerated in certain conditions (Table 3.2). Resting tremors that continue during posture and movement arise usually from lesions in the brain stem region of the red nucleus (rubral lesions). Sometimes a Parkinsonian tremor is still evident in posture and movement. Instruments are available

Table 3.1 Definitions of 'neurological' movement disorders

Tremor	An involuntary continuous rhythmic oscillation of a body member
Tics	Purposeless, stereotyped, repetitive, jerking movements, that can be voluntarily suppressed at the expense of increased psychic tension
Chorea	Irregularly-timed jerking movements of varying distribution
Myoclonus	Brief shock-like muscular jerks
Dystonia	Sustained or clonic muscular spasm distorting part of the body
Athetosis	Slow, irregular, writhing movements, most frequently starting in the fingers and toes
Hemi-ballismus	Unilateral, intermittent, coarse, jumping movements of the limbs

Table 3.2 Causes of tremor

Static/rest tremor	Extrapyramidal disorders e.g. Parkinsonism

Postural tremor	'Benign' essential tremor
	Parkinson's/structural brain disease
	Physiological tremor — exaggerated by
	   Emotional arousal (anxiety/stress)
	   Thyrotoxicosis
	   Alcohol withdrawal
	   Withdrawal of beta-blockers
	   Drugs (sympathomimetics, lithium,
	   amitriptyline, caffeine)
	Flapping tremor

Intention tremor	Cerebellar or brain stem disorder

for the measurement and recording of tremor, and may assist in diagnosis.

A Parkinsonian tremor may be accompanied by the other features of Parkinsonism — cogwheel rigidity and bradykinesia with immobile facies and shuffling or festinent gait and a flexed posture. Parkinson's disease is liable to be misdiagnosed as retarded depression, if the accompanying rigidity and tremor are not detected. Because an exaggerated physiological tremor is common in anxiety, it is important to remember that there may be other causes (see Table 3.2), and that an essential tremor may affect particular occupational or leisure activities (writer's tremor, vocal tremor etc).

Intention tremor is best demonstrated by the finger-nose test for upper limbs and the heel-shin test for lower limbs. It is indicative of cerebellar or brain stem disorder, and associated signs include nystagmus, ataxia and clumsiness of rapid alternating movements, e.g. tapping movements of the hand or foot, or the touching of the thumb with each finger in succession. The occurrence of ataxia with confusional symptoms should alert the doctor to the possibility of Wernicke's encephalopathy, and indicates further examination for nystagmus, extrinsic ocular palsy, and peripheral neuropathy. This diagnosis is one of the most urgent in psychiatry because of the severe disability that results from a delay in treatment (Korsakov's syndrome). Common causes of cerebellar intention tremor include multiple sclerosis and phenytoin intoxication. Wilson's disease is among the rarer causes.

Hysterical tremor

Hysterical tremor occurs either as an exaggeration of physiological tremor with additional jerking movements. or as a resting and postural tremor at the natural resonant frequency of the limb or head; the result resembles a Parkinsonian tremor, but other aspects of Parkinsonism are lacking.

TICS

Tics are common in childhood, especially in boys, and usually last only a few weeks or months. They involve mainly the face and head, and their most common form is blinking. They are exaggerated by emotional upset. There is often a family history of tics. They are more likely to become chronic if they have attracted excessive attention in a tense, obsessional child. However, a small proportion of cases develop multiple tics and some of these go on to develop other features of Gilles de la Tourette's syndrome — vocal tics or explosive word utterances which may be grunts or swear words (coprolalia), and echolalia. Most of these persons have normal intelligence and no mental disorder but the social consequences of the condition may badly affect them. Tics also result from drugs or following encephalitis. When they develop in adulthood (usually after age 40) they tend to be limited to a single muscle group and to run a chronic course.

CHOREA (Table 3.3)

Huntington's chorea is an autosomal dominant disorder which does not usually present typical symptoms until adulthood, although prior to the presentation of chorea, there may be a variety of psychiatric symptoms including severe depression, suicide attempts and personality disorders. The manifestations are a combination of progressive chorea and dementia. Widespread choreiform movements occur, which the patient disguises by making them seem intentional. Patients have a characteristic facial appearance with a wide-eyed stare and wrinkled brow. A laboratory diagnosis of Huntington's chorea may soon be possible using the G8 gene probe as a genetic marker.

Table 3.3 Causes of chorea

Huntington's chorea	
Hereditary chorea	
Sydenham's chorea	
Drug-induced	Anti-psychotic drugs
	Dopamine agonists, L-dopa and
	amphetamines
	Phenytoin
	Anti-cholinergics
Symptomatic	S.L.E.
	Thyrotoxicosis
	Encephalitis
	Hypoxia
	Hypernatraemia
	Hypercalcaemia

Table 3.4 Some causes of dystonia

Drug-induced dystonia	
	Acute dystonia
	Tardive dystonia
Tardive dyskinesia	
Primary focal dystonia	
	e.g. Spasmodic torticollis
	'Occupational' cramps
	Blepharospasm
Symptomatic secondary dystonias	
	e.g. Cerebral palsy
	Wilson's disease
	Lesch-Nyhan disease
	Juvenile Huntington's
	disease
	Post-encephalitic
Primary familial dystonias (*dominant, recessive, X-linked or sporadic*)	
	Dystonia musculorum
	deformans
	Paroxysmal dystonia.

Other hereditary choreas may be dominantly inherited but commence in childhood and are not accompanied by severe psychiatric disorders. Sydenham's chorea is the consequence of rheumatic fever (now rare in Britain) and develops in childhood after a streptococcal infection. The chorea may recur during pregnancy or when the contraceptive pill is taken.

MYCLONUS

Myoclonus may occur in normal people whilst in bed at night. It also occurs in association with a number of uncommon neurological disorders often accompanied by fits, in metabolic and toxic disorders and occasionally with generalized idiopathic epilepsy. It may occur in Alzheimer's disease, Jakob-Creutzfeldt disease, uraemia, hepatic failure, respiratory failure, hyponatraemia, hypocalcamia and alcohol withdrawal. The EEG helps in determining the aetiology and planning further investigations for metabolic disorders.

In hemifacial spasm there are irregular shock-like contractions of one side of the face. The condition continues for many years, and ipsilateral facial weakness develops. It is caused by pressure on the facial nerve, usually by local blood vessels.

DYSTONIA

Some of the causes of dystonia are shown in Table 3.4. Although primary and drug-induced cases are more common, dystonia can be symptomatic of a large number of organic brain diseases and metabolic diseases.

Acute dystonic reactions occur frequently during the early stage of treatment with antipsychotic medication, particularly in young people (see Table 3.5). The commonest presentations are those affecting the tongue, eyes, or a limb. An oculogyric attack consists of fixed upward deviation of the eyes, and is often accompanied by dystonia of the tongue and increased salivation. Alternatively a bizarre gait may result from dystonia of a lower limb. Torticollis may also occur. Because this reaction occurs in psychiatric patients it is liable to be misdiagnosed as a hysterical conversion symptom, malingering, or even as epilepsy or tetanus, with embarrassing results. Even an improvement in response to suggestion or to a placebo is no confirmation of an hysterical basis for the symptoms, because drug-induced dystonia will sometimes improve too. Other substances that may cause acute dystonias are metoclopramide, dopamine agonists, anticonvulsants and manganese.

The term tardive dystonia refers to the occurrence of dystonia in patients who have received antipsychotic medication for a long period of time — usually two to three years. Young males are most likely to be affected. The condition persists after discontinuation of medication and may represent the precipitation of primary dystonia. The condition is more disabling than tardive dyskinesia.

Tardive dyskinesia

Tardive dyskinesia is the term used to describe the delayed occurrence of a range of abnormal movements in patients on antipsychotic drugs. The phenomenon is thought to represent hypersensitivity of dopamine-receptive neurones, owing to prolonged blockade of dopamine receptors. The condition is worsened by anticholinergic drugs and may improve temporarily with an increase in the dose of antipsychotic medication. The commonest syndrome of tardive dyskinesia is orofacial dyskinesia (oro-bucco- lingual-masticatory syndrome) in which there occur chewing and lip-smacking movements and the tongue moves into the cheeks or in and out of the mouth ('fly-catcher tongue'). Less commonly the limbs or trunk show abnormal writhing (athetoid) or choreiform movements. Dopamine agonists including amphetamines and L-dopa can produce similar dyskinesias. There is controversy about the extent to which tardive dyskinesia is caused rather than exacerbated by drugs. Similar movements occur spontaneously in older people, and those with dentures, and in unmedicated chronic schizophrenics. Tardive dyskinesia is more common in the elderly, in females, in patients with other forms of organic brain disease (e.g. a history of head injury) and in patients who have developed Parkinsonism earlier in the course of treatment with antipsychotic drugs.

Primary focal dystonias

Spasmodic torticollis is a repetitive involuntary turning of the neck due to spasm of the muscles of the neck, especially of the sternomastoid, which usually starts at 30–45 years of age. A few cases may be hereditary. Although emotional factors may worsen it, the condition is now thought to have a mainly organic basis. An hysterical form of torticollis may be distinguished by the lack of true spasm of muscles, by the absence of any other abnormal movements and sometimes by the presence of a recognizable depression or other psychiatric disturbance.

Blepharospasm arises from spasm of the orbicularis oculi muscles. It may precede the development of Parkinsonism or other dystonic symptoms. It should not be confused with excessive blinking which is a feature of some forms of schizophrenia, or which may occur as a tic in some individuals under stress.

Occupational 'cramps' are rare focal dystonias affecting particular complex movements, while sparing other movements that involve the same muscles. In writer's cramp the dystonia affects the fingers and other parts of the limbs during writing. Although it has an organic basis it can be modified by psychological factors and some cases are best regarded as psychosomatic.

Secondary (symptomatic) dystonias

As well as drugs there are a number of other physical causes of dystonias. These include brain damage following perinatal trauma or kernicterus, head injury, encephalitis, or anoxia; and a number of rare genetic disorders of metabolism including Wilson's disease, Lesch-Nyhan disease and Juvenile Huntington's disease. A careful history and examination needs to be supplemented by a variety of specialist neurological investigations.

In Wilson's disease, disorder of copper metabolism leads to lesions in the basal ganglia. The psychiatric complications include a schizophrenia-like syndrome. Serum copper, caeruloplasmin and 24-hour urinary copper levels are abnormal. There is a brown Kaiser-Fleischer ring in the cornea.

Lesch-Nyhan disease causes mental retardation, with dystonia and self-mutilatory acts. Xanthine-oxidase deficiency is responsible. When Huntington's disease presents in adolescence it produces dystonia and an akinetic-rigid syndrome. Hemidystonia, affecting the limbs on one side of the body, is sometimes due to a space-occupying lesion or infarct of the contralateral basal ganglia which can be recognized on the CAT scan.

ATHETOSIS

Athetosis may take various forms but most commonly affects the limbs, trunk and face. It may be a sequel of kernicterus, or result from perinatal hypoxic brain damage or haemorrhage. The degree of mental retardation may be quite unrelated to the severity of the athetosis. After kernicterus, there may also be high-tone deafness which can result in a misleading underestimation of mental ability.

HEMIBALLISMUS

Hemiballismus results from lesions of a small area of the brain associated with the subthalamic nucleus.

DRUG-INDUCED INVOLUNTARY MOVEMENTS (Table 3.5)

The drugs most incriminated are the dopamine-receptor blocking agents used for their antipsychotic effect. Other dopamine-receptor blocking drugs such as metoclopramide may also cause some of the same syndromes. Other antipsychotic drugs such as reserpine, which acts by depleting dopamine stores, produce some but not all the movement disorders. Some of the characteristics of the syndromes are shown in Table 3.5. The incidence of these side-effects depends upon the drug used, and is highest for dystonias and Parkinsonism in those drugs lacking intrinsic anticholinergic activity (haloperidol, pimozide, etc). Sometimes the side-effect is seen more with low doses than with higher doses and it may occur a few days after medication has been discontinued, when blood levels of the drug have fallen.

Acute dystonia, tardive dystonia and tardive dyskinesia have already been considered. Drug-induced Parkinsonism resembles idiopathic Parkinson's disease except that the rest tremor is less prominent. It is important to observe the posture and movements of psychiatric patients before they are treated with antipsychotic drugs, for sometimes they already show abnormalities that could easily be mistaken subsequently for the side-effects of medication.

Akathisia is an inability to keep still, with a subjective sense of restlessness and unease, and a particular tendency to shift from foot to foot. The subjective experience may be mistaken for anxiety due to the underlying psychiatric disorder. Anticholinergic drugs are only partially effective in counteracting akathisia.

Certain antipsychotic drugs have been found to produce a form of catatonia (see below), characterized by muscular rigidity with waxy flexibility. This may be related to the even more severe and dangerous condition of the neuroleptic malignant syndrome in which muscular rigidity is accompanied by pyrexia and leucocytosis.

ABNORMAL VOLUNTARY MOVEMENT

Abnormal voluntary movements are defined in Table 3.6. Although all these may occur in catatonia, which is discussed below, combinations of these phenomena may also occur in non-catatonic schizophrenia, organic brain disease, mental handicap and other psychiatric and physical conditions. In untreated schizophrenia there may be a variety

Table 3.5 Drug-induced movement disorders

Name of disorder	Time of onset	Incidence	Age predominance	Response to anticholinergic medication
Acute dystonia	1–4 days	3–10%	Young adult	+
Akathisia	10–90 days	10–20%	None	+/0
Parkinsonism	14–90 days	10–20%	Middle age and elderly	+
Tardive dyskinesia	$\frac{1}{2}$–3 years	10–20%	Elderly	−
Tardive dystonia	2–3 years	Uncommon	Young male	+/0
Catatonia	Days	Rare	None	0
Neuroleptic malignant syndrome	Days	Rare	None	0

+ Improves
0 No influence
− Worsens

Table 3.6 Definition of abnormal voluntary movements

Stereotypy	a repetitive purposeless act or utterance carried out in a uniform way.
Mannerism	a purposeful act that is consistently carried out in a strange way, that may be idiosyncratic or may be an imitation of someone. For instance the patient may shake hands with two fingers, or may copy the gestures of someone well-known.
Perseveration	the senseless repetition of a goal-directed action when it is no longer appropriate. For instance the patient repeats the answer to a previous question, or continues to carry out an act previously required of him.
Echopraxia	the copying by the patient of movements made by someone nearby.
Automatic obedience	the carrying out of all instructions, regardless of the consequences.

Table 3.7 Catatonic phenomena

Movements	Speech
Stereotypies	Stereotypies
Mannerisms	Manneristic voice
Grimacing	Neologisms
Automatic obedience	Verbigeration
Echopraxia	Echolalia
Perseveration	*Vorbeireden* (talking past the point)
Catalepsy	Perseveration
Waxy flexibility	
Mitgehen	
Co-operation (*Mitmachen*)	
Opposition	
Negativism	
Obstruction	
Ambitendency	

of abnormal spontaneous and induced movements. The abnormal spontaneous movements include an increased blink rate, sterotypies, tics, and mannerisms. Abnormal induced movements in schizophrenia include perseveration, automatic obedience and echo-phenomena. Sometimes the movements resemble tardive dyskinesia with tongue protrusion, writhing of the hands and grimacing. Some of the abnormal movements occur early in the course of schizophrenia, but others seem to develop particularly when the patient is kept for a long period of time out of a normal social environment, either at home (desocialization) or in hospital (institutionalization).

Organic brain disease affecting the frontal lobes can lead to perseveration and automatic obedience, for instance in dementia. In mental handicap there is also a tendency to develop stereotypies, including rocking, head-banging and tics. Again institutionalization and desocialization contribute to this.

CATATONIA

The term catatonia is used to refer to a variety of abnormalities of posture, movement and speech. The symptoms seem to indicate abnormalities of volitional control of the neuromuscular apparatus. Catatonia is a syndrome rather than a diagnosis.

Table 3.7 shows the varied symptoms of catatonia. Stereotyped postures include *Schnauzkrampf* — pouting in which the protruded lips resemble a snout — and 'psychological pillow' — the patients lie with their heads a few inches above the pillow and maintain this for a considerable period. Catalepsy is when the patient maintains for long periods postures which have been imposed on them by examiner, although told that they do not have to do so. When this happens, and the examiner has a feeling of plastic resistance when moving the patient's limbs, it is called waxy flexibility (cf cataplexy, chapter 5). *Mitgehen* is an extreme form of co-operation (*Mitmachen*) in which the slightest pressure from the examiner will move the patient's body in the direction of the pressure, even though the patient is told to resist this.

Opposition is the resistance by the patient to all passive movements, of whatever force. Negativism is an apparently motiveless resistance to suggestions or interference; active negativism is when the patient does the opposite of what is asked, in a reflex way. These must be distinguished from the motivated non-cooperation of the stubborn or hostile personality. Obstruction is the sudden block of co-operative movement; this may result in 'reaction at the last moment': e.g. the patient fails to respond until the examiner stops questioning. Obstruction differs from depressive psychomotor retardation by its inconsistency, but both phenomena can lead to stupor (see below). Ambitendency is a manifestation of obstruction or negativism in which the patient makes tentative movements in accordance with the examiner but does not complete them.

Catatonia is associated with abnormalities of speech that may be regarded as mannerisms (see chapter 11). Other features of catatonia will be discussed below under stupor and excitement.

The occurrence of catatonic symptoms should not lead to a diagnosis of schizophrenia unless there is other more specific evidence of that condition, such as the first-rank symptoms of Schneider (see chapter 17) or abnormalities of affect and association. Isolated catatonic symptoms especially mannerisms are common in mania. Catalepsy may occur in hysterical dissociative states. In addition to frontal lobe brain damage, other neurological and metabolic disorders can produce symptoms of catatonia, such as catalepsy (see Table 3.8). The EEG may be useful in discriminating between organic and functional causes of catatonia. Florid catatonic states are seen less frequently than in the past, and are now most likely to occur in psychotic patients with a foreign language or culture.

Table 3.8 Causes of catatonia

Psychiatric	
	Schizophrenia
	Manic-depressive illness
	Dissociative states
Neurological	
	Basal ganglia lesions
	Temporal lobe lesions
	Space-occupying lesions of the IIIrd ventricle
	Encephalitis
Metabolic disorders	
	e.g. hypercalcaemia
Toxic disorders	
	Psychostimulants e.g. amphetamine
Drugs	
	Antipsychotic agents e.g. fluphenazine decanoate

STUPOR

Stupor is a state of complete psychomotor inhibition (absence of speech and movement) with retention of consciousness. As well as muteness and lack of movement, there may be failure to feed spontaneously, and incontinence. There is a risk of dehydration, venous thrombosis, pulmonary embolism, chest infection, and ulceration of skin and pressure areas. In partial stupor there is a limited amount of movement and speech. Table 3.9 shows the types of stupor.

In depressive stupor there may be a history of gradually increasing retardation. The facies appear depressed. There may be some diurnal variation in the degree of stupor. The patient may show more response to questioning on less emotive topics.

In catatonic stupor the patient shows, together with the features of stupor, one or more of the symptoms of catatonia, in particular stereotyped postures and catalepsy. In catatonic states due to schizophrenia, there may also be evidence of affective incongruity with unexplained rage or laughter, and pronounced negativism. Also in catatonic schizophrenia there may be sudden changes from stupor to excitement; during the excitement there may be evidence of thought disorder with neologisms. The patient may also eat voraciously during the excitement phase, having neglected to eat during stupor. The EEG is often abnormal in catatonic stupor, and the epileptic threshold is lower. Urinary incontinence is common and faecal incontinence may occur in this form of stupor. Responsiveness to pain may be absent.

Psychogenic stupor occurs after a severe fright when the patient may remain speechless and immobile for a time. Hysterical stupor may occur as a prolongation of a response to a shock, and there may then be evidence of some secondary

Table 3.9 Types of stupor

Depressive stupor
Catatonic stupor
Manic stupor
Psychogenic stupor
Organic stupor

Table 3.10 Organic stupor — causes

Neurological
Tumour in IIIrd ventricle (cyst etc)
Midbrain lesions — Craniopharyngioma
                    Pinealoma
                    Basilar aneurysm
                    Trauma
                    Encephalitis
Temporal lobe epilepsy
Petit mal epilepsy

Toxic/metabolic
Carbon monoxide poisoning
Hypothyroidism
Hyperparathyroidism
Hypoglycaemia
Hepatic encephalopathy
Uraemic encephalopathy
Lithium intoxication
Neuroleptic intoxication

gain. In malingering, patients tend to eat when unobserved, and this may be suspected when the patient maintains a well-hydrated appearance while refusing offers of food or fluid. Manic stupor is a form of mixed affective disorder in which retardation of speech and movement is accompanied by elation of mood; catalepsy may also occur.

The causes of organic stupor are shown in Table 3.10. Cases due to lesions of the midbrain may be called 'akinetic mutism'. Investigations in cases of stupor should include EEG, blood tests and in certain cases lumbar puncture (when raised intracranial pressure is ruled out and tumour is not suspected). Fluid balance charts and regular checking of temperature, pulse and blood pressure are needed. Information of diagnostic value may sometimes be obtained in stuporose patients from the response to a slow intravenous injection of diazepam or amytal to produce light sedation. Sometimes the patients will then accept food. Often the patient will talk more freely and his thought content may aid diagnosis; schizophrenic patients may reveal delusional ideas and hallucinations, or formal thought disorder, whereas depressed patients may express morbid thoughts. Cases of psychogenic stupor may remain improved after an initial abreaction following the injection.

CASE HISTORY

JOHN FRANKLIN

John Franklin was the 21-year-old youngest son in a family who reluctantly agreed to a domiciliary visit by a psychiatrist. He lived at home with his 60-year-old mother, his unmarried sister of 41 and a divorced brother of 30. There were two other married siblings who lived away from home. John's father had died suddenly of a myocardial infarct eighteen months previously at the age of 65.

Mrs Franklin consulted her GP because she was worried about John, although he himself had no complaints. She said that for about a couple of weeks John had been quiet, withdrawn, had lost his appetite and seemed preoccupied. He had developed a habit of looking nervously over his shoulder when he was walking around the house, and she heard him up and about during the night. She had become alarmed the previous night when she was awakened by a crash of china in the kitchen and had gone downstairs to find John shaking, sobbing, and staring fixedly at the corner cupboard. He would not say what was wrong.

The domiciliary assessment was difficult because of the family's extreme embarrassment at John's condition; his oldest sister tried to introduce the psychiatrist as a friend. John sat fixedly in a chair, darting sideways glances at his family, and with an anxious posture; he was hunched over and he gripped his hands tightly together. He made no reply when asked what was wrong, and could not be encouraged to speak at all until his mother and siblings left him alone with the doctor. He then, in a quiet, low voice, answered in monosyllables and had no spontaneous speech. He admitted he felt frightened and 'wrong', but was unable to explain in what way. On direct questioning he agreed that he had been sleeping badly and that the previous night in the kitchen he thought there was someone there with him, although when he turned to look, he could see no one. He said that he thought he heard someone talking, although he did not know what they were saying. He admitted that this had happened several times in the last two weeks, but he could explain it no further. Once or twice during the interview he screwed his face into a wide grimace, without an explanation. He also gazed all round the room during the conversation and obviously had difficulty in concentrating. His mood was one of bewilderment, although he said he was sometimes sad. He was not retarded and there was no objective evidence of depression.

Further history was obtained from his mother and sister. His mother claimed he had done quite well at school and had made friends. Since leaving school five years before, he had worked for a year in a supermarket filling shelves. He had left this job after coming home in tears because the manager had told him he was too slow. Since then he had not attempted to find another job, but had helped around the house, taken his dog for walks and watched television. He had no friends and made no attempt at a social life, but it was clear that this was not viewed as a problem by the rest of the family who were obviously equally isolated socially. Mrs Franklin said that John had got on well with his father and had been upset when he died but no one in the family had talked about him much after the funeral so she could not say whether he was still grieving. There was a family history of psychiatric illness in that Mr Franklin's sister had spent the last 40 years in a psychiatric hospital, having been admitted at the age of 23; no further details were available.

John shook his head when asked if he would consent to a hospital admission, and his mother absolutely refused to consider the idea. Fortyeight hours later, however, Mrs Franklin rang in distress to say that John seemed very ill. He had been found in his underwear, standing immobile in the street outside, and it had been difficult to encourage him to return to the house. He had not said a word after this, and had not eaten anything, although he would drink if his mother held the cup. She said that he seemed frightened and would stare for long periods of time into the corner of the room, although he also smiled and laughed from time to time.

On reassessment, John's mental state had changed. He was standing on one foot in his bedroom and did not acknowledge the arrival of the psychiatrist and his mother. When asked to sit down he did so, but stood again quite quickly and then resisted his mother's attempts to push him towards the chair. He raised his arm when asked to shake hands, but did not complete the movement. When the psychiatrist scratched his own head, he did the same, and copied several other movements made by the doctor. He maintained his arm in the air, when it was placed there by doctor, for over a minute, although told he could put his hand down by his side. He was completely mute.

Questions

What is the likely diagnosis of John's condition?
What investigations are necessary?
What are the immediate risks?

John is in stupor; he is mute and immobile. Several features indicate that this is catatonic — he demonstrates both negativism and automatic obedience at different times, shows echopraxia, and waxy flexibility has been clearly elicited. His grimacing in the initial interview — and possibly his reported smiles and laughter — is also catatonic movement. He shows no speech abnormalities at this stage.

The cause of this catatonic stupor is not certain, but schizophrenia must be the likely diagnosis. Although his family minimize his difficulties, it is clear that John has been abnormally introspective and withdrawn for some time. He was probably responding to auditory hallucinations when the incident occurred in the kitchen; and had been suspicious and afraid of people whom he could not see behind him for some days. His affect is flat — not overtly depressed. There is a family history of probable severe mental illness, although clarification is needed on this point.

There is no evidence, from either the history or the mental state examination, that this stupor is depressive. An organic cause to the catatonia must however, be ruled out. A full physical examination is required, although he is unlikely to be able to co-operate in a comprehensive neurological examination. Haematological and biochemical screening should be carried out. Any evidence of a focal brain lesion must be fully investigated as must any sign of an infectious illness. An EEG is important, since although it is often abnormal in catatonic states of any cause, it is necessary to exlude encephalitis, which produces characteristic and severe disruption of the EEG, in which frequent, non-focal slow waves are seen.

The immediate risks are twofold: firstly that John will become dehydrated, and secondly that his stupor will give way to a phase of excitement. It has been difficult for Mrs Franklin to persuade John to drink, and he will eat nothing — his fluid intake must be monitored. If it becomes imposs-ible to keep him hydrated by mouth, intravenous hydration might be attempted, although it is doubtful that he would tolerate this procedure.

As soon as an organic cause has been excluded, treatment with major tranquillizers should be commenced with a view to relieving his stupor as quickly as possible. If dehydration becomes a reality, electroconvulsive therapy is indicated. Catatonic excitement states can develop very quickly and without warning in patients such as John; this is potentially dangerous both to himself and to his family, who may be harmed by unpre-meditated and motiveless aggression in such a context.

These risks are sufficient indicators of the need to admit John to hospital compulsorily, even in the face of continued opposition from his family.

4

Eating disorders

In the investigation of suspected eating disorders, the difference between hunger, appetite, food consumption and weight must be borne in mind (See Table 4.1). The links between them are obvious; the assessment of which aspect is primarily disturbed is sometimes difficult, but always important. Hunger and appetite are not identical phenomena although their differences are masked in communities where there is insufficient food, and hunger, malnutrition and low weight prevail. In most Western countries food is widely, probably excessively, available, and the differences become more pronounced. Hunger is an internal cue that food intake is required and the cue is dependent on physiological needs as well as learnt behaviour, such as feeling hungry at lunch time. Appetite, however, is much more dependent on non-physiological factors such as the sight, smell and anticipation of food. This principle underlies most of the snack food advertising prevalent in Western urban culture.

Eating habits and weight maintenance are profoundly affected by social expectation, in countries where food is not scarce, and minor variations are most appropriately viewed as a social, rather than a medical, concern. The current Western preoccupation with thinness as a desirable goal leads to eating and exercise behaviour which would have been considered abnormal only forty years ago.

The aspect of eating most important in a psychiatric sense is appetite and its effect on the relationship between food consumed and energy expended. Weight loss in the face of normal appetite and food intake indicates a systemic organic cause such as malignant disease or tuberculosis. While diminished appetite together with weight loss may be a sign of primary physical illness, psychiatric causes are also prominent. Lesions in hunger and satiety centres in the hypothalamus are rare causes of profound weight change, dependent on hunger and its satisfaction rather

Table 4.1 Some differences in the relationship between appetite and weight

	Hunger	Appetite	Weight
physical illness such as 1 *carcinoma*	decreased	decreased	decreased
2 *thyrotoxicosis*	increased	increased	decreased
Depressive psychosis	decreased	decreased	decreased
Milder depression	no change	unchanged decreased increased	no change mildly decreased increased
Anxiety	no change	increased/decreased	increased/decreased
Hypothalamic lesions	{ increased { decreased		increased } decreased }
Anorexia nervosa	no change	no change	decreased
Bulimia nervosa	no change	periods of increase	increase & decrease

than the external psychological and social triggers of appetite.

Patients, however, rarely present with a complaint of appetite change, but rather with a problem concerning weight. The important feature is any change from the previous norm; and a careful history of the onset of the problem, eating patterns and a record of weight change are essential in the assessment of all such patients.

DISORDERS ASSOCIATED WITH REDUCED APPETITE/WEIGHT

DEPRESSION

The differential diagnosis depends on the age of the patient, in addition to other features of the history and mental state. In middle-aged and elderly patients, severe anorexia and weight loss is most commonly due to a depressive illness. The extent and speed of weight loss is indicative of the severity of the depression. Minor depression of mood causes a transient appetite disturbance which may not result in any appreciable weight loss, but a severe depression may produce weight loss of more than a stone in a few weeks. A patient thus affected will have other biological signs of a severe depression, such as sleep disturbance, loss of energy and slowing of thought and action. He may or may not complain of depression of mood. He will admit that his appetite has disappeared and that his food intake is drastically reduced, but will frequently not volunteer this as a problem. His attitude, rather, may be that he has lost interest in food and, importantly, in the necessity to eat correctly in order to stay alive and well. Statements such as, 'I can't eat' should not be taken at face value but investigated more thoroughly, since they may divulge underlying depressive delusions. Severely depressed patients may have nihilistic delusions (Cotard's syndrome) (see chapter 14). Such delusions frequently centre around eating and patients may believe that their stomach is full of stones, that their bowels have rotted, that they cannot break down food and so on. Depression causes perceptual change too, and complaints that food has lost its taste or tastes bad may be elicited. Severely depressed patients do not feel hungry, and have no appetite. They may

be convinced that this is due to a physical lesion and request investigation although it is more commonly a matter of complete lack of interest to them.

The pattern of history and mental state should not provide a diagnostic problem, but it must be remembered that serious physical illness may itself present as depression, especially in middle-aged and elderly patients. Thorough physical examination and appropriate investigation must always be carried out. Malignant disease, especially metastatic or hormone-producing, may underlie the entire problem and should not be forgotten in the assessment of the patient who is depressed, cachectic and ill, especially in the absence of previous personal or family history of affective psychosis.

Other psychotic illness

Patients suffering from mania may lose weight because they are so busy with their multiplicity of exciting plans and schemes that they cannot be bothered to eat, rather as they cannot find time to rest and sleep. They will ignore feelings of hunger or eat erratically and inappropriately. Untreated manic patients may collapse from exhaustion, and inadequate nutrition contributes to this. They rarely, however, escape notice long enough for serious weight loss to result.

Weight loss may occur in both acute and chronic schizophrenia. Acute paranoid schizophrenics may be deluded about their food, believing that it is poisoned or contaminated in some way. Patients may avoid specific foods or food prepared by specific people, but appetite *per se* is not affected.

Chronic schizophrenic patients may fail to eat normally as part of a general inability to care for themselves. There is usually no problem when such patients are cared for by others at home or in hospital, but if living on their own, patients chronically disabled by schizophrenia may not have sufficient drive or ability to buy, prepare and eat an adequate diet.

Demented patients living alone may become malnourished in similar ways although the cause here is more specific. Demented patients forget how to prepare food and forget meal times.

Anxiety states may be associated with reduced appetite, although many anxious people eat more, or more sweet and 'comforting' foods. When anxiety operates to lower appetite, weight loss is usually mild and gradual and is not a major complaint.

ANOREXIA NERVOSA

In younger patients who are losing weight, anorexia nervosa must be considered in a differential diagnosis. This is primarily a condition of adolescent or young adult women but since 10 to 15 per cent of cases occur in males the diagnosis must also be considered in men. Despite its name, anorexia nervosa is not a disorder of appetite and affected patients will not present with this complaint. They rarely present spontaneously at all but may be brought by an anxious parent. Patients may complain of unexplained weight loss but frequently deny that anything is wrong. If a careful and reliable history of eating habits and attitude to food is not obtained, unnecessary and mistaken investigations for systemic disease may be undertaken. The diagnosis of anorexia nervosa depends on establishing a pattern of food, and therefore weight, avoidance — often in the face of maintained appetite and hunger. The central symptoms are twofold: firstly the wish to remain thin and prepubertal in physical development, and secondly the need to establish control of appetites, of which food intake is but one. Amenorrhoea, primary or secondary, is the rule, and although to be expected as the body responds to starvation, may occur before weight has fallen to critical levels and may even precede the weight loss. Severely malnourished patients may have dependent oedema due to hypoproteinaemia and are at risk of circulatory collapse.

The eating pattern in this condition is remarkably constant. Patients will specifically avoid carbohydrate foods, which they perceive as fattening, and will eat as little they can, for example one apple and a yoghurt a day, despite all attempts to persuade them to eat more. They will often find it impossible to eat with others and will eat apart from their family. Food becomes the major focus of family life, and apparently paradoxically, the patient may devote much time and energy to cooking for the family whilst declining to eat herself. This activity is partly to test out and reinforce her feeling of security in controlling her appetite for food. The disorder is allied to the fear of losing control of other appetites, specifically sexual, and invariably reflects serious underlying abnormalities in family relationships, especially between mother and daughter.

A typical history from an anorexic patient reveals that food was a battleground between mother and daughter in infancy — food fads, temper tantrums around meal times and anxiety in the mother about the child's nutritional status are common. Many anorexic girls are overweight before the illness begins, decide to diet, and then apparently cannot stop when they reach a normal weight. Whether the condition begins after dieting or whether the onset of anorexia is initially taken for normal adolescent female concern with slimness is unresolved.

The other area of family relationships which is frequently disturbed is that between the patient and her brothers and sisters. Usually the patient tells of longstanding problems of jealousy, envy and feelings of inferiority between her and, most commonly, an older sister. She will feel she is less attractive, less clever, less accomplished and less loved. In some cases it becomes apparent that being ill is the only thing she feels better at than her sister, and thus the only way to obtain a greater degree of love and concern from the family.

Other features in the history may include enthusiastic, often excessive, exercising to the point of exhaustion; and further attempts to reduce weight by vomiting and by the consumption of purgatives (see below).

The mental state of the anorexic patient can be difficult to assess at first if she is a reluctant uncooperative patient, steadfastly denying that anything is wrong. Her appearance will usually reveal her excessive thinness, especially on the face, but her body may be hidden by layers of bulky clothing so that the full extent of her weight loss is not apparent. Patients often look younger than their years. She will appear sullen, denying, calm and uninterested. Alternatively she may be unhappy, bewildered and ashamed. Once sufficient trust is established, she will reveal how miserable and worried she is and usually reveal a greater degree of insight into her condition than was immediately apparent. Thought content in these patients is overwhelmingly about self-control, food, and weight, the patient confessing that she spends time naked in front of a mirror estimating her weight, and that she daydreams of plans about her food intake. It is common to find that she is emphatic in her belief that she is fat, despite evidence to the contrary, and this clinical finding is in line with the research evidence that disordered body image is frequent.

Physical examination

A thorough physical examination is mandatory for all patients in whom anorexia nervosa is suspected. The patient's weight (undressed) and height should be recorded on a chart which indicates percentiles for height and weight. The patient will be noticeably, sometimes extremely, thin, with loss of muscle bulk and wasting. Peripheral circulation may be poor and dependent oedema resulting from low serum protein may be present in severe cases. The distribution of body hair is normal but there may be soft, downy hair (lanugo) on the arms and face. Evidence of the consequences of malnutrition, such as vitamin deficiency or pneumonia, may be identified.

Investigations

Dehydration may result in raised urea and an artefactually normal haemoglobin although iron deficiency anaemia occurs. Electrolyte disturbances result from vomiting and purgation, of which alkalosis and hypokalaemia are the most important. Hormonal abnormalities reflect the hypothalamic-pituitary dysfunction. Plasma cortisol and growth hormone levels are increased, and luteinizing hormone is reduced.

The differential diagnosis is rarely difficult if enquiry is directed to attitudes about the food and weight rather than leaving the patient's statement that she eats normally unexplored. It is rare for anorexia nervosa to begin after the establishment of satisfactory sexual and reproductive life, but an underlying undiagnosed anorexic problem may be revealed upon marriage or childbirth and this

needs careful elucidation. Severe depressive illness should be ruled out after the history and examination. In older texts, Sheehan's syndrome (panhypo-pituitarism as a result of postpartum infarction) is noted as an important differential diagnosis, but this rare condition has almost nothing in common with anorexia nervosa, except for secondary amenorrhoea.

It is at the milder end of the spectrum that diagnostic difficulties occur and this is therefore a greater problem in general than in psychiatric practice. The discrimination between early anorexia nervosa and appropriate concern with body image in normal adolescence may be difficult, especially where menstrual regularity is poorly established. Careful monitoring of weight over time is indicated and many of these cases are self-limiting or are revealed as problems in over-anxious mothers who are too uncritical of what they read in the press or see on television.

Boys with anorexia nervosa are rarely seen. The clinical picture is very similar with a failure of sexual development together with diminished food intake. They are usually even more disturbed in their psychosexual development than affected girls, and their prognosis, in terms of establishing satisfactory adult heterosexual relationships, is worse.

DISORDERS ASSOCIATED WITH INCREASED APPETITE AND/OR WEIGHT

Obesity is a major health problem of overindulged affluent countries. Mild obesity is a social rather than a medical concern and its definition is dependent on fashion rather than physical factors. Gross obesity presents cardiovascular, respiratory and musculoskeletal problems and shortens life expectancy.

The vast majority of grossly obese subjects eat high calorie foods consistently to excess. However the relationship between obesity and overeating is not simple, since there is a great variety in energy expenditure between and within persons; and many individuals who eat a lot are not overweight. Interest is current in energy expenditure, genetic predisposition and fat metabolism in the grossly obese which may validate the claims of some of the many obese patients that they, 'Eat like a sparrow, Doctor'. Diaries of all obese subjects demonstrate that they eat much more than they believe, however, and there is evidence that obese people are much more cued by appetite and habit than by hunger.

Most obese patients do not have definable psychiatric conditions. Most, however, report that they eat more 'comfort' foods when lonely and unhappy, with the argument that in the absence of anyone else to indulge, or to be indulged by, they will indulge themselves. Women who are depressed and isolated with husband and children away from home frequently turn to the kitchen fridge for support. Obesity is embarrassing at best and repulsive at worst so that the consequent shame and rejection perpetuates a vicious circle. Clear-cut psychiatric conditions are, however, sometimes associated. Occasionally patients who are clinically depressed overeat, although this is confined to the milder depressions. Some overweight people develop depressive illnesses when they attempt to diet and this phenomenon, which may have physiological as well as psychological causes, makes continued dieting difficult. Anxiety increases appetite in as many people as it decreases it, and some patients gain and lose weight as their anxiety states fluctuate.

OTHER EATING DISORDERS

Some people have eating disorders whilst maintaining a normal weight or a widely varying abnormal weight. Studies of women in the general population have shown that a significant minority have intermittent problems in weight control, using combinations of dieting, overeating in uncontrolled bouts (binge-eating) and self-induced vomiting. For some this behaviour is linked to stresses and life events, but only a few see it as a problem requiring medical help. Patients who do present for help have a severe disturbance of eating behaviour although their weight is usually within normal limits. The characteristic pattern is of rigid dietary control, interrupted by bingeing which is either planned or spontaneous and may involve the consumption of vast amounts of food. Bingeing is distinguished from 'normal' overeating because it is experienced by the individual as being out of control, is at first intensely pleasurable although subsequently guilt-producing, and is secretive. Bingeing is then followed by self-induced vomiting. Some patients vomit after every meal as well after binges. Purgative abuse is common.

In recent years this condition has been classified as a separate entity: *bulimia nervosa*. It is clear, however, that its psychopathology is markedly similar to that of anorexia nervosa and it can be seen as an extension of that condition, insofar as the fear of anorexics that eating will become out of control has been acted out in reality by patients with bulimia. A previous diagnosis of anorexia nervosa can be made for about half of those currently suffering from bulimia nervosa. However, some differences have emerged: bulimia nervosa is almost exclusively confined to women, and the

Table 4.2 Comparison of anorexia Nervosa and bulimia nervosa

	Anorexia nervosa	Bulimia nervosa
Sex distribution	80% female	Almost exclusively female
Age of onset (typical)	14–25	14–40
Weight maintained	normal to low	normal to high
Premorbid weight	normal to high	high
Menstruation	1° or 2° amenorrhoea	Amenorrhoea or irregular menses
Central problem	fear of fatness	fear of fatness
Weight controlled by	dieting (+ exercise) vomiting & purging	dieting, vomiting & purging
Serious medical complications	starvation, circulatory collapse	hypokalaemia dehydration gastric dilatation

age of onset falls within a wider range, up to forty years. In addition these women are rarely thin, they are less evasive about the condition and they reveal a greater level of depression and anxiety than anorexic patients (see Table 4.2).

Bulimia nervosa has severe physiological consequences. Binge-eating can be so extreme that acute, potentially fatal gastric dilation can result. Vomiting and purging severely disrupt metabolism and chronic hypokalaemia with the risk of cardiac arrhythmia is often found, together with other problems of dehydration, paraesthaesia and tetany. Purgative abuse leads to steatorrhea and frequent vomiting erodes tooth enamel. The event which finally persuades the patient to seek help may be the realization that her teeth are wearing away or her fillings are falling out.

There should be no diagnostic difficulty with this group of patients. Depression and anxiety are secondary to the problem which, like anorexia, centres around the fear of becoming fat. Some patients have learnt to vomit spontaneously and the self-induced character may not immediately be apparent; however, no physical illness combines frequent vomiting with eating of this type, with its secretive, sexualized, ritualistic quality.

FUNCTIONAL (PSYCHOGENIC) VOMITING

Self-induced vomiting is almost always indicative of anorexia nervosa or bulimia, but occasionally patients are referred whose only symptom is repeated vomiting over which they have no control. This is usually a variant of the above conditions whereby vomiting has become automatic, uncontrolled and feared, but sometimes there is no evidence from the history or mental state to support either diagnosis. Vomiting of this type is related to anxiety, either generalized or phobic; it may be an attention-seeking or manipulative symptom or, rarely, a hysterical conversion.

CRAVINGS OF PREGNANCY

There may be superficial behavioural similarities to bulimia nervosa especially when hyperemesis is present, although the phenomenology is quite different. Cravings usually occur in the first and second trimester, and are usually specific for a particular type of food or flavour. They are usually self-limiting and transient and do not lead to major disturbance. Their origin is unknown but thought to be a combination of psychological and physiological causes: both a somewhat regressive search for comfort and a result of altered perception of taste and smell in pregnancy.

CASE HISTORY

JANE CARPENTER

Jane, a 23-year-old woman, was seen at home at the request of her GP who said he thought she was suffering from depression. Jane was in her dressing-gown in the mid-afternoon, looked pale and cold, was slowed down in speech and action, sat for long periods silently staring into space and answered questions with the minimum of words. She was tall, with long blonde hair in need of washing, and was obviously thin. She complained of depression of mood so that she could see no fun or joy in living and admitted that she was both eating and sleeping poorly.

Her boyfriend, with she had lived for about a year, confirmed a marked change in mood over the last three or four months, so that Jane had become miserable and unresponsive, complained of feeling ill and had cancelled several social appointments: for example, to go to friends for dinner. She had first attended her GP about two weeks before when she had felt unable to go to work and since then she had sat at home, crying on occasion but refusing to talk either to him or to her family. He was particularly worried because she would not eat and became angry with him when he pressed her to.

At this point Jane interrupted him and said she was eating but did not like to be bullied about it. She said she ate when he was out at work but he disputed this. She claimed to eat cereals for breakfast, soup for lunch and to eat a proper evening meal. She agreed that her appetite was diminished and that she had lost weight. She did not know how much — her boy friend said it was a great deal, particularly since she was already thin, having been concerned to keep her weight down ever since he had known her. He said, for example, that although she used to cook for him and when entertaining friends, she hardly ever ate a complete meal.

He thought that her condition had deteriorated about the time, four or five months ago, when she had failed to become promoted at work; she was in advertising and had achieved well, expecting promotion to a senior position in the firm, and had been surprised and upset when the post was given to a colleague. She admitted that her confidence had been shaken by this.

They both claimed a good relationship and said it was a stable, long term one, although they did not envisage getting marrried in the near future. Their sexual life was described as satisfactory to both, and Jane, who was on oral contraception, said she had normal monthly periods.

Jane was the middle child of three — she had a sister aged 28 and a brother aged 21. Her father was a successful businessman in good health, although he had been given ECT during a psychiatric admission ten years before at the age of 45, and had been extensively investigated for physical illness during a period of weakness and lethargy three years ago. Jane described an affectionate, although undemonstrative relationship with him; she was much closer to her mother, who did not work, was described as providing an exceptionally close and warm home for her children and was still interested and concerned about them. She rang Jane frequently and often asked her to spend the weekend at home. It became clear that this was a problem between Jane and her boyfriend: Jane's parents knew of their relationship but did not know that they were living together and the couple quarrelled about Jane's insistence on deceiving them because she said they would be hurt and would not understand. Jane was fond of her brother and sister although she saw them only at her parents' house. Her brother was living at home at present since he had taken a year off from university; six months before he had had psychiatric day hospital treatment for depression and it had been decided that he should retake his second year.

Jane said her previous life was free of difficulty and she remembered a happy home. She was good at school, made friends easily, and had had no

difficulties in her childhood. Her only setback was failure to gain admission to Cambridge where her elder sister had succeeded. She had no previous psychiatric or medical history.

Physical examination revealed Jane to be thin with evidence of peripheral vasoconstriction. No other physical abnormality was detected. She was five feet eight inches (1.73 m) tall and weighed seven stone, eight pounds (49 kg). Biochemical and haematiological investigations were normal except for a haemoglobin of 10.8 g/dl, a serum iron of 10 μmol/l and a total iron binding capacity of 70 μmol/l.

Questions

What is the differential diagnosis of Jane's condition? What further information is required to confirm it?

The differential diagnosis lies between anorexia nervosa and a major depressive illness. Neither diagnosis is, at this stage, absolutely clear-cut and if a diagnosis of anorexia nervosa is to be sustained, one must assume that Jane is dissimulating, as suggested by her boyfriend.

She is profoundly underweight for her height and has a (nutritional?) iron deficiency anaemia which indicates an inadequate diet for longer than three months. We do not know whether or not she has amenorrhoea since she is on oral contraception which will produce withdrawal bleeding. It appears that she has a chronic concern with slimness which has been kept within normal limits but in recent months she has lost a great deal of weight although she denies abnormal intake. Against a diagnosis of anorexia nervosa is the absence of previous difficulties and the fact that she has established an apparently successful adult sexual relationship. In addition, she is not claiming to be overweight or admitting to any phobia or guilt about food intake. There is, however, evidence that she avoids eating in public.

She is undoubtedly markedly depressed, unable to work or to carry on a normal social life, with evidence of psychomotor retardation and sleep disturbance. The issue is whether her condition is primarily depressive or secondary to anorexia nervosa. Her weight loss is profound and if depression were the cause of this one would expect other depressive symptoms to approach it in severity. Most notably, Jane does not complain of a decrease in appetite sufficient to cause this degree of weight loss. She has, however, a strong family history of psychiatric illness and it appears that both her father and her brother have suffered from depression.

A third possibility is that Jane is suffering from a physical condition causing her anaemia, weight loss and depression. Her prominent complaint is of a nonspecific malaise. There is no evidence of this on investigation or on examination but the possibility must be borne in mind.

There are several areas from which more information must be derived before the diagnosis can be confirmed. Firstly Jane's actual eating pattern and response to food must be observed for evidence of food, especially carbohydrate, avoidance, or vomiting after meals and to ascertain her attitude to her weight. Her mood, including diurnal variation and sleep pattern, is important. Much more needs to be known about her current and past relationships; the pattern of her relationships with men; previous sexual relationships which she has had, if any; her attitude to her current relationship and her hopes and fears about it and whether or not she wants children. It is important to interview her family so that a fuller picture of her early and adolescent life emerges and it will be very useful to see Jane and her mother together to observe the nature of their relationship. Finally, details of the psychiatric illnesses of her father and brother should be obtained.

There are strong hints from her initial interview that anorexia nervosa is the likely diagnosis: a picture emerges of a studious, friendly, 'good' girl, close to her mother but not to her father or siblings, who remains very attached to her parents and dependent on their approval. She cannot tell them the nature of her relationship with her boyfriend for fear of their disapproval but neither can she solve the conflict by marrying; perhaps because the commitment is too daunting. She has career ambitions but failed (in competition with her sister?) to achieve Cambridge entry and her recent relative failure at work may have precipitated an acute exacerbation of anorexia nervosa; it may, on the other hand, have precipitated a depressive illness. Her mother may reveal evidence of childhood food fads and anorexic behaviour in adolescence.

It is possible that upon full assessment the diagnosis will be of two conditions — firstly a chronic anorexia which she has controlled in the past without treatment but which has worsened with the conflicts surrounding her first serious sexual relationship; and secondly the added recent development of a depressive illness, to which she is genetically predisposed, triggered by her loss of self-esteem and confidence after failing to achieve the job she wanted.

5

Sleep

Although dreams have been a major concern of psychoanalysis since its development at the beginning of this century it is the last twenty years that have seen the development of physiological interest in sleep disturbances. Research into normal and abnormal sleep has increased greatly with the establishment of sophisticated sleep laboratories enabling the diagnosis of such disorders as narcolepsy and sleep apnoea syndrome, in patients previously labelled as hysterics or malingerers. The pharmacotherapy of sleep has progressed with the development of safer and short-acting hypnotics though these bring with them the potential hazard of over-prescribing.

Epidemiological surveys have shown that around a third of the population are dissatisfied with the amount or quality of their sleep. There is a wide range of normal periods of sleep. Anything between 4–10 hours a night is probably within normal limits and the length of sleep decreases with age. Differences within individuals are more meaningful than those between them.

Why we sleep remains largely an unanswered question. It may be related, at least in children, to growth hormone secretion, and circadian rhythms govern much of our internal body functions. Sleep deprivation produces a markedly abnormal mental state with altered perception and ideation, and reduced psychomotor skills.

PHYSIOLOGY OF SLEEP

Normal sleep as recorded by electroencephalography is of two types, non-rapid eye movement (NREM) and rapid eye movement (REM).

NREM sleep is made up of four stages through which the normal person passes sequentially, stage one being the lightest and stage four the deepest. The electroencephalogram (EEG) in NREM sleep shows generalized slowing, especially in stages three and four with sleep spindles and K complexes. REM sleep is characterized by decreased muscular activity as measured by the electromyogram (EMG) apart from the ocular muscles which show rapid eye movements. The EEG shows marked brain activity and penile erections occur during this phase. This is the time when people dream and if the patient is woken up during REM sleep he can often give details of his dreams.

In the normal person, sleep cycles start with NREM sleep from stages one to four lasting about 1–1½ hours followed by REM sleep lasting 5–10 minutes. The cycle is repeated 4–6 times a night with the REM sleep lasting progressively longer in each cycle and representing all together some 20–25 per cent of the total night's sleep. The percentage of REM sleep decreases through childhood; with ageing there is an increase in light sleep (stages one and two) with a corresponding decrease in deep sleep (stages three and four), and sleep may frequently be interrupted.

NEUROCHEMISTRY, NEUROENDO-CRINOLOGY AND NEUROANATOMY

5-hydroxytryptamine, noradrenaline and acetylcholine have all been implicated as neurotransmitters governing sleep and dopamine has been associated with waking behaviour. Growth hormone secretion peaks during sleep throughout childhood and adolescence, and prolactin is also secreted during sleep. Anatomically, sleep appears to be mediated through the brain stem.

ASSESSMENT OF SLEEP

Many patients present with symptoms suggestive of sleep disturbance; as with any presenting symptom it is important to take a full history and mental state, and, where relevant, make a physical examination. It is especially important to clarify what the patient means by sleep disturbance. Is it quantitative or qualitative? Is excess sleep being confused with episodes of daydreaming, escape into fantasy life, failure to concentrate or transient changes in levels of consciousness as in epileptic phenomena? In sleep impairment, is the patient really complaining of tiredness and lack of energy and drive regardless of the number of hours slept? An informant, such as the spouse, may be best placed to give an objective assessment of the patient's sleep. Sleep charts may help to delineate the pattern of sleep. If doubt remains, the patient may need to be admitted to hospital for an objective evaluation, though not infrequently the patient will deny having slept at a time when the nursing staff say he slept well. The patient's answer to this may be that he has been lying on his bed with his eyes closed but not asleep. If all else fails the EEG can be monitored continuously in a sleep laboratory.

SLEEP DIFFICULTIES

Patients may complain of too little sleep — difficulty getting off to sleep, disturbed nights, waking early or a combination of the above; too much sleep; or a reversed sleep pattern — sleeping during the day and not at night. There may be episodes of sleep walking or talking, restless legs in bed, hypnagogic or hypnopompic hallucinations, nocturnal enuresis or bruxism. Dreams may be disturbing as in nightmares, night terrors may occur; patients may occasionally complain that they have stopped dreaming or spent the whole night dreaming.

Table 5.1 Causes of insomnia

1 *Physical symptoms* — pain, breathlessness, nocturia, cramp

2 *Physical illness* — CNS disorders including delirium

3 *Psychiatric disorder* — mood disturbance

4 *Drugs* — stimulants, excess daytime sedation, sedative withdrawal, drug toxicity

5 *Central or diaphragmatic sleep apnoea*

6 *Restless legs syndrome*

7 *Idiopathic*

Insomnia (see Table 5.1)

The causes of this are manifold but need to be accurately determined if sleep is to be improved. Of particular interest in psychiatry is sleep impairment as the result of psychiatric illness or its treatment. Anxiety tends to cause difficulty in getting off to sleep or waking during the night, whereas severe depression is often associated with early morning waking and being unable to get off to sleep again. Mania is associated with sleeping very little if at all. Psychotropic medication may interfere with sleep in a number of ways (see Table 5.2). Sleep impairment may be caused by drugs with stimulant properties, and by commonly used substances such as coffee and excess alcohol. In addition, drug toxicity may lead to acute confusional states with reversal of sleep pattern; sedation during the day may relieve the need to sleep at night; and withdrawal of hypnotics, including alcohol, induces a temporary alteration of NREM/REM pattern with associated sleep disturbance. Fifteen per cent of people complaining of insomnia are said to be suffering from insomnia with no identifiable cause. Some patients who complain of being unable to sleep can be shown under laboratory conditions to sleep for normal periods of time. It is clear from this that sleep as a subjective experience may be different from its objective observation.

Lethargy

Some patients say that they have not slept deeply and feel tired on waking. This is usually a

Table 5.2 Effects of drugs on sleep

	Total sleep time	Number of awakenings	Sleep latency	REM	SWS
Benzodiazepines	↑	↓	↓	–	↓
Barbiturates	↑	↓	↓	↓	↓
Phenothiazines	↑	–	↓	–	↑
Tricyclic antidepressants	–	↓	–	↓	↑
Monoamine oxidase inhibitors	–	–	–	↓	–
Amphetamines	↓	↑	↑	↓	↓
Lithium	↑	–	–	↓	↑
Alcohol	↓	↑	↓	↓	↓

↑ increase
– does not affect
↓ decrease
SWS = Slow Wave Sleep

Berrios, G. E. (1982). Sleep and its disorders. In: *Readings in Psychiatry*, p.52, The MEDICINE Publishing Foundation, Oxford.

complaint of lethargy, often associated with affective disorders, rather than of true insomnia. Neurasthenia was a fashionable diagnosis for people complaining of nervous exhaustion though it is now accepted that this is usually associated with depression and anxiety. Lethargy may also be due to organic disease, e.g. myxoedema, Addison's disease or cardiac failure. It may be confused with the apathy seen in chronic schizophrenia or the loss of interest of severe depression.

Restless legs

Two rare syndromes in which insomnia occurs are central or diaphragmatic sleep apnoea (see below) and restless legs.

This consists of a crawling sensation in the legs, only relieved by moving them, which leads to considerable interruption of sleep. It may be associated with nocturnal myoclonus, which may also occur alone in which a rhythmic jerking of the limbs occurs which sometimes wakes the person.

Hypersomnia (see Table 5.3)

Patients may complain of sleeping for longer hours than usual, drowsiness during the day or sudden attacks of sleepiness. Excess sleep may be physio-

Table 5.3 Causes of hypersomnia

1 Physiological	— post-sleep deprivation
2 Physical	— structural CNS lesions — metabolic disorders
3 Psychiatric	— stupors — hysterical states
4 Narcolepsy	
5 Sleep apnoea (Pickwickian syndrome)	
6 Kleine-Levin syndrome	
7 Idiopathic (sleep drunkenness)	

logical, psychological or pathological. It may be due to cerebral disorder following structural lesions in the midbrain or hypothalamus, the latter associated with excess hunger and weight increase, or to disturbances of metabolism. In these cases sleep tends to be sustained, undisturbed and not refreshing. Psychiatric disorders may lead to a complaint of hypersomnia as in the case of hysterical disorders, or may be confused with it in psychotic stupors. It may be drug-induced, whether by sedatives or alcohol, or part of a number of specific syndromes.

Narcolepsy

Narcolepsy is characterized by the presence of some or all of the following four symptoms: excessive sleepiness, usually occurring as sudden bouts of sleep often associated with severe drowsiness in between attacks; cataplexy which is loss of muscle tone and control often leading to falls, usually precipitated by emotional arousal; sleep paralysis; and hypnagogic hallucinations. These hallucinations, commonly in the auditory modality, although sometimes visual and tactile in nature, occur during the transitional period from waking to sleep and more rarely from sleep to wakefulness when they are called hypnopompic. There is often disturbed nocturnal sleep. Narcolepsy may occur in isolation but may be associated with psychiatric disorders such as depression and schizophrenia.

Onset is usually around the age of puberty and there is sometimes a family history. Patients with narcolepsy tend to go spontaneously into REM sleep without passing through a non-REM stage and the EEG during cataplexy shows a REM-like picture. The attacks of sleep occur when the person is not tired, sometimes in inappropriate and dangerous circumstances, as while driving a car.

Sleep apnoea syndrome

This syndrome consists of episodes of respiratory impairment during sleep and is of three types: diaphragmatic or central apnoea, where the diaphragm stops moving during sleep; obstructive or upper airways sleep apnoea where the upper airways become obstructed; and a mixture of the two. Upper airways sleep apnoea is associated with loud snoring and abnormal body movements, moaning and groaning and sleepwalking; there may be many hundreds of apnoeic episodes each night. It may occur during non-REM sleep only, during REM and non-REM sleep, or during REM sleep and transitional stages. These patients suffer from severe daytime sleepiness as opposed to those with a central or diaphragmatic sleep apnoea which is usually associated with insomnia. Other abnormalities associated with this syndrome are hypertension, nocturnal hypoxia and nocturnal cardiac arrhythmias. It is often found in obese people when it may be called the Pickwickian syndrome but may also be found in people of normal weight.

Kleine-Levin syndrome

This disorder usually occurs in young men and consists of periodic episodes of sleepiness associated with intense hunger, irritability, excitement and aggression, together with disturbances of movement, thinking and perception. Each episode may last from days to weeks with long periods of normal sleep in between, although the episodes may be followed by depression and insomnia.

Sleep drunkenness (Idiopathic hypersomnolence)

Patients with this disorder may have difficulty in waking up completely and this is associated with confusion, disorientation, poor motor co-ordination, slowness, repeated return to sleep with long periods of sleep and usually, daytime sleepiness. It has its onset in childhood or young adulthood and occurs more commonly in males than in females. It is sometimes seen in families and there may be associated psychological disturbances.

Reversed sleep pattern

Patients with acute confusional states suffer from clouding of consciousness, and are drowsy during the day but show increased arousal at night when their behaviour is often most disturbed. Other disturbances of sleep pattern include jet-lag, where the individual has difficulty adjusting to a new time zone, and phase lag and phase lead syndromes where the patient sleeps and wakes late or early.

Table 5.4 Parasomnia

Sleepwalking (somnambulism)

Sleeptalking

Night terrors

Nightmares

Nocturnal enuresis

Bruxism

PARASOMNIAS (SEE TABLE 5.4)

These are disturbances of behaviour which occur during sleep.

Sleepwalking (somnambulism)

Sleepwalking consists of stereotyped, repetitive and purposeless movements which occur while the patient is asleep, when he may answer questions monosyllabically and may be suggestible. Somnambulism usually lasts for minutes although in some cases it may last a half hour or more. It is due to partial arousal from sleep during the non-REM stage of sleep and is more frequent during the first third of the night when sleep is at its deepest. It is most common in children, especially in males, and there may be a family history. It is associated with enuresis; and in adults, with psychiatric disorders. Sleeptalking may be associated with sleepwalking and, like the latter, it is commoner in males and occurs during the deep stage of non-REM sleep.

Night terrors

These are brief episodes of raised arousal with anxiety, screams and increased autonomic nervous system activity occurring during non-REM sleep in stage three or four. It is often associated with sleepwalking and is commonest in children, but when it occurs in adults it may be associated with psychiatric disorders. In contrast to nightmares which occur during REM sleep, night terrors occur during non-REM sleep.

Nocturnal enuresis

Though most children become dry day and night from the age of two to three years, a decreasing small percentage remains wet, especially at night time, and this sometimes continues into adulthood. Nocturnal enuresis is commoner in boys and its aetiology is multifactorial with anatomical, pathological, psychosocial and possibly genetic contributions. It may be primary, in which case the child has never been dry; or secondary, when it occurs after a period of established proper bladder control. When nocturnal enuresis develops secondarily it frequently follows a period of stress or disruption in the family or in the child's routine.

Bruxism

This is nocturnal grinding of the teeth which may lead to wear and tends to occur during light sleep, stages one and two. Its aetiology is unknown. It is sometimes a cause of persistent facial pain due to strain on the temporomandibular joint.

CASE HISTORY

MRS JEFFERSON

Mrs Jefferson, a 54-year-old widow, attended psychiatric out-patients at her own request. She complained of anxiety, depression and insomnia of about eighteen months' duration. She said that she felt fed up, couldn't get interested in her housework or anything else and became restless at home; she spent most days out, either wandering around the shops or visiting one or other of her neighbours. She complained particularly bitterly of the insomnia, saying that she had always been a poor sleeper but in recent months had had many nights when she had not slept at all, and that she could not remember when she had last had an undisturbed night's sleep.

There was no consistent pattern to her sleeplessness; usually she would go to bed around midnight and fall asleep without much difficulty. She would wake after an hour or two of sleep and sometimes was able to fall asleep again immediately but more often she lay in bed awake for a further hour or two. She would then get up and have a cup of tea and a cigarette, returning to bed in the early hours of the morning. Sometimes she then slept for two or three hours but frequently, recently, did not sleep again, with the result that her final waking time was around two a.m. Whatever the pattern of her night's sleep she awoke unrefreshed and felt irritable. She usually got up to prepare breakfast for her family, and would do her housework, but in recent weeks her household tasks had interested her less and she performed them desultorily. Some mornings she would doze off over a cup of tea and do little, if anything.

Mrs Jefferson had become increasingly uncomfortable and unhappy in the house where she felt tense and guilty. She sometimes felt that she had to get out of the house. This feeling was only present when she was alone.

Her early history was unremarkable; she was the third and last child of a warehouse packer and his wife, and had experienced a close and happy family life. One sister survived whom Mrs Jefferson saw every couple of months; this sister had married 'well' and lived to a substantially higher standard than the patient. There was no family history of psychiatric illness.

Mrs Jefferson had been an indifferent scholar; she had left school at fourteen and worked in a factory until her first pregnancy, since when she had not worked. She had become engaged at nineteen to her first serious boyfriend, had married at twenty-two and had three children, daughters now aged 30 and 21 and a son of 24. Her husband, a local authority manual worker, had, like Mrs Jefferson, been quiet, homeloving and content without an active social life apart from regular family contact. Mrs Jefferson had been an active, good mother and housekeeper, and was proud of her role as carer for her and her husband's parents as they aged and died. She had developed no interests and few social contacts outside the home.

Seven years before, Mr Jefferson had died suddenly and unexpectedly at the age of 52 of a myocardial infarct. Mrs Jefferson had grieved actively for about a year, had been well supported by her children and her other family and believed she had overcome her loss, 'as far as it is possible — I still miss him sometimes'. Her older daughter had left home to be married at the age of 25 and visited Mrs Jefferson about once a fortnight. Her other two children were living at home, both working and both enjoying an active social life, leaving her alone most evenings. Her daughter had a steady boyfriend and talked of marriage in the future, and Mrs Jefferson said, 'children aren't what they were — they don't tell their parents much — don't respect them like we did in my day'.

Direct questioning revealed Mrs Jefferson had suffered from chronic bronchitis and emphysema for many years. She had taken benzodiazepine tranquillizers by day and hypnotics at night since her husband's death and felt that they weren't strong enough. She smoked 30 cigarettes a day, and admitted to drinking alcohol — whisky — at night to help her sleep, but said that she rarely had more than two drinks. She also said that for the last year of two she had been visiting the local club with a female neighbour a couple of nights a week, where she drank stout.

Examination of Mrs Jefferson's mental state revealed a woman of low normal intelligence, cognitively intact, whose mood was depressed, but who established reasonable rapport, and was spontaneous, with no evidence of psychomotor retardation. She denied suicidal ideas but said that the future seemed dull and lonely; such that though she would not dream of harming herself she wouldn't mind much if she developed a fatal illness. She was not anxious, but somewhat sullen and hostile.

Her younger daughter, who was interviewed separately, said that her mother had changed over the last three years from a helpful, usually cheerful and supportive mother to a miserable, irritable and critical person. As a result, Mrs Jefferson's son had become somewhat estranged, was less helpful in the house and brought his friends home infrequently. She confirmed her own plans to marry in about a year's time. Most significantly she said that all the children were very worried by their Mother's alcohol intake; she found empty whisky bottles quite frequently, thought that her mother was drinking about half a bottle of whisky a day and that in the last couple of months she had been drinking before the children returned home from work. She had found her drunk on a few occasions and said that before her father died, neither parent drank often: both were infrequent, minimal social drinkers. Mrs Jefferson's daughter also said that three weeks before, her aunt, who did not drink, had visited and had a row with her mother over the amount she was drinking.

Questions

What is the significance of the insomnia?
How should this be treated?
Mrs Jefferson has a mixed anxiety and depressive condition which is moderate in severity. She is unhappy and pessimistic and feels that life is not

enjoyable or fulfilling, and she is aware of anxiety and worry throughout most of the day. It is important to decide whether the insomnia is caused by depression, since if it is, this is the most positive evidence of the presence of a major depressive disorder; there is little else in the history or mental state to indicate that depressive illness is the primary problem. The biggest problem is Mrs Jefferson's increasing use of alcohol; she is, for the first time in her life, drinking regularly to excess and she is hiding the quantity she drinks. Although she claims to be using alcohol as a hypnotic, her sleeplessness has worsened as her intake has increased and it is likely that the alcohol is contributing to the insomnia. There remains a possibility that her relatively recent earlier wakening is depressive, but it may also be due to alcohol abuse, which in turn may be masking an anxiety-related initial insomnia. Both these points will be clarified on her response to treatment.

The insomnia is also significant because it is Mrs Jefferson's main complaint and to encourage her compliance with treatment of the whole condition, attention must be given to relieving her most troublesome symptom, not least because she feels it is sleeplessness which results in her drinking.

The complete treatment plan will depend on her response to the early stages. She must be encouraged to relinquish both the alcohol and, subsequently, the benzodiazepines. Her sister and her children should be enlisted to support her, and care should be taken that she is not further isolated by the removal of her only social contact- the club. It may be appropriate to suggest that she aims to stop drinking whisky, but that she can drink a couple of stouts at the club with her friend two or three times a week. She needs to be warned that her sleep will get worse whilst she withdraws from drugs — inability to tolerate this may indicate admission for inpatient treatment. The long term treatment plan must include helping Mrs Jefferson to find a new role in life as her children leave home — she should be helped to the realization that encouraging them to stay with her because she needs them will cause unhappiness to all in the long term. Mrs Jefferson's ability to find enough interests, hobbies and feeling of worth outside the immediate family will determine her long term prognosis. Antidepressant medication is not indicated at this stage; if, however, depressive symptoms become apparent during treatment, it may become necessary.

6

Sexual disorders

DEFINITION

Sexual dysfunction is a term used for difficulties with normal heterosexual pratice.

Sexual deviation is defined as sexual behaviour occurring in other than the normal heterosexual setting. This rigid definition obviously leads to difficulties when considering homosexuality and masturbation.

TAKING A SEXUAL HISTORY

This is often the most difficult part of the psychiatric history, engendering embarrassment for both the interviewer and the patient. To some extent this explains why sexual problems are sometimes presented indirectly with other physical symptoms such as headache, which are more acceptable and easier to talk about. It may not be possible to ask in detail about sexual aspects of the history in the first interview, especially when the patient has not come complaining directly of sexual problems. In these cases it is important to record what has not been asked, so that this can be dealt with in subsequent interviews when the patient feels more at his/her ease. The sexual history should be dealt with tactfully, and if necessary, euphemisms such as physical relationships may need to be used. One should start by assessing the age at which puberty occurred and in women this should include menstrual history. This provides the interviewer with a relatively natural introduction to the later, potentially more embarrassing, topics of sexual contact.

The sexual history should include the following areas:

1 psychosexual relationships, age at which they develop and any problems
2 engagements or marriages and other steady relationships
3 children
4 sexual activity including masturbation, age of onset, fantasies and any masturbatory guilt, heterosexual and homosexual feelings and behaviour, and where relevant, deviant sexual behaviour

It is important to enquire into the expectations of the patient as these may not be realistic; for example, the man who presents with impotence because he is only able to have intercourse three times a night rather than the ten times which he feels is normal. Any change in sexual behaviour, and its precipitating causes, is important.

When patients present with sexual problems it is important to make a detailed behavioural analysis of their sexual habits in order to ascertain clearly the nature of the patient's complaints. Both the attitude of the patient to sexual behaviour and his/her level of sexual knowledge should be determined. After interviewing the patient it is important to take an independent history from the partner and to see the couple together. This may take more than one interview and it is useful for the patient to fill in a diary of sexual activity in between appointments.

SEXUAL DYSFUNCTION

This can be divided into the following subgroups depending on where, in the sexual act, the disturbance lies.

	Male	*Female*
i Desire	low libido	low libido
ii Arousal	erectile impotence	failure of arousal
iii Orgasm	premature ejaculation retarded ejaculation	orgasmic dysfunction
iv Pain	on ejaculation	vaginismus dyspareunia

Adapted from Gelder, F. M., Gath, D. and Mayou, R. (1983). *Oxford Textbook of Psychiatry*. Oxford University Press.

Terminology

Men

Erectile impotence is the inability to develop or sustain an erection. This may be partial or complete, temporary or permanent, primary or secondary (depending on whether erection has ever been normal). Premature ejaculation is ejaculation either prior to penetration or very soon after, whereas retarded ejaculation is delay or failure to ejaculate, usually during intercourse.

Women

Failure of arousal includes failure of vaginal lubrication and orgasmic dysfunction is absence of orgasm. Vaginismus is muscular spasm of the vagina causing tightness and pain on attempted penetration whereas dyspareunia is pain on intercourse. The term frigidity is unhelpful as it does not state where in the sexual act the disorder lies.

Normal sexual function

Normal sexual activity usually commences sometime after puberty, and is probably most frequent at the onset of steady relationships, e.g. marriage, after which it declines in frequency and reaches a plateau. A further decline in frequency occurs either gradually with increasing age, though there is no upper age limit for full sexual activity, or acutely, following a physical or psychological stress. There are sometimes short periods when sexual activity is less frequent than at other times. Sexual activity may occur either in the setting of a stable relationship or as part of a shortlived, sometimes financial, relationship. Though monogamy is the socially accepted form of behaviour in Western society in some cultures it is considered normal practice for one man to have many female sexual partners and more rarely, for women to be polyandrous.

Control of sexual function

In both males and females normal sexual function is under the control of physiological mechanisms. Sexual drive — libido — is to some extent controlled by hormones. An increase in androgens is associated with the increase in sexual drive seen in males at puberty, and if females are given small doses of androgens their sexual drive also increases. Psychological factors are important in sexual drive.

Arousal and orgasm are under the control of both central and peripheral neurological mechanisms. Erection in the male is mediated by erectile centres in the sacral and thoracolumbar parts of the spinal cord which act via parasympathetic and sympathetic nerves respectively, and which are influenced by central pathways in the brain. Ejaculation is mediated by sympathetic nerves from the lumbar part of the cord and motor nerves from the sacral part. As with erection, ejaculation is also influenced by the brain. In women the neurological control is probably similar to that in the male with genital lubrication and swelling in the female corresponding to erection in the male, and orgasm in the female to ejaculation.

Epidemiology

In males the most frequently presented complaint of sexual dysfunction is impotence. This increases with age up to the level of almost one in five by the age of sixty. In female patients lack of sexual enjoyment is the commonest problem.

Aetiology

Sexual dysfunction may be organic or psychological in origin (see Tables 6.1 to 6.3).

Desire

Lowered libido

Though this may sometimes be due to endocrine disorders it is most commonly psychological in origin and associated with personality difficulties and relationship discord.

Arousal

Erectile impotence

This is the male sexual disorder where organic factors are most likely to be relevant (see Table 6.4). Despite this it is still most likely to be due to psychological factors including performance anxiety, relationship discord, fear of exacerbating coexisting illness and fear of pregnancy and commitment. It is also sometimes seen following traumatic accidents even where there has been little organic damage, possibly related to alteration

Table 6.1 Aetiology of sexual dysfunction in people with physical illness

Physical illness	
Endocrine	— diabetes, hypogonadism, adrenal cortical failure, pituitary disease, thyroid disorders.
Cardiovascular	— ischaemic heart disease, microvascular.
Neurological	— spinal cord damage, brain injury.
Arthritis	
Respiratory	— asthma, chronic obstructive airways disease.
Local genital disorders	— penile and vaginal lesions, pelvic inflammatory disease, endometriosis, ovarian lesions.
Renal	— renal failure.
Following surgery	
Gynaecological	— hysterectomy, oophorectomy, carcinoma of the uterus, vaginal repair for prolapse, episiotomy.
Abdominal and pelvic	— colostomy, ileostomy.
Prostatectomy	
Amputation	
Psychological reaction to physical disorders	
Altered body image	
Anxiety about harm or pain	
Fear of failure	
Post-operative depression	
Partner's anxiety or rejection	
Poor medical communication	
Anxiety about sexual activity in pregnancy	

Medication (see Table 6.2)

Table 6.3 Psychosocial causes of sexual dysfunction

Sexual ignorance

Personality difficulties

Relationship discord

Lack of a partner

Poor self-image

Fear of commitment

Fatigue

Fear of damaging the partner

Fear of damaging oneself

Fear of failure — performance anxiety

Fear of pregnancy

Mood disorder

Environmental factors

Table 6.4 Organic causes of impotence

1	*Neurological*	autonomic neuropathy — diabetes spinal cord damage brain damage — temporal lobe tumours of IIIrd ventricle
2	*Cardiovascular*	Leriche syndrome
3	*Local genital pathology*	priapism, congenital malformations, prostatectomy
4	*Endocrine disorders*	Primary and secondary hypogonadism testicular atropy — cirrhosis — haemachromatosis — dystrophia myotonica — other causes
5	*Alcohol*	
6	*Drugs* — (*see* Table 6.2)	

in self-image. Organic impotence can be differentiated from psychogenic impotence by the fact that the latter is often situational; for example, it may only occur during coitus or with a particular partner whereas early morning erections and masturbation may be unaffected. Temporary impotence is common and usually self-limiting.

Failure of arousal in women may also be organic in nature but is much more commonly due to psychological factors.

Orgasm

Men

Premature ejaculation is rarely organic in nature but is often associated with anxiety. Total inability to ejaculate may be organic due to neurological disturbance or drugs, but when it only occurs in a specific situation, for example in intercourse, it is psychologically caused and suggests underlying psychosexual difficulties.

Women

Anorgasmia Although total anorgasmia may be due to physical factors, many women who are both physically and psychologically normal never have an orgasm. Women are more dependent than men on tactile stimuli for arousal and many women reach pre-orgasmic states of arousal much more slowly than men. Many anorgasmic women are only in the initial stages of arousal when inter-

course is completed. Failure to achieve orgasm is thus commonly the result of poor communication between partners, ignorance of the significance of sexual foreplay and anxiety in the male partner. It may well be that the increasing attention focused in this area is a product of the media's representation of 'normal' sexual habits putting pressure on anorgasmic women and making them feel failures. This may produce psychosexual problems where none had previously existed.

Pain associated with sexual behaviour

Pain in the penis

This may occur during erection or ejaculation or even outside the sexual act. Except in cases of organic pathology this is due to psychological factors including psychosexual personality difficulties, depression, hysterical conversion neurosis or anxiety states.

Pain in the female genitalia

This can be divided into vaginismus and dyspareunia. Except in cases where vaginismus acts to prevent penetration which would be associated with pain due to local physical pathology, it is almost always psychological in nature and associated with marked anxiety about sex.

Dyspareunia — pain on intercourse — on the

Table 6.2 Effects of medication on sexuality

Drug	Probable mechanism of action				Likely effects on sexual response		
	Central	Sympathetic blockade	Para-sympathetic blockade	Other	Desire	Excitement	Orgasm
Anticholinergic Probanthine			+			May cause impotence	
Antidepressants Tricyclics			+			May cause impotence	Possible delayed ejaculation
MAOI's			+			May cause impotence	Possible delayed ejaculation
Antihypertensives i Central-acting Methyldopa		+			Reduced	May cause impotence	May be inhibited
ii Ganglion blockers Hexamethonium Mecamylamine		+	+			May cause impotence	May cause failure of ejaculation or retrograde ejaculation
iii Alpha-blockers Clonidine		+					Emission may be inhibited
iv Beta-blockers Propranolol	+	+			May be reduced	May cause impotence	
v Adrenergic blockers Guanethidine Bethanidine		+				Often cause impotence	May cause failure of ejaculation or retrograde ejaculation
Anti-inflammatory	+				May be reduced		
Indomethacin Anti-Parkinsonism L-dopa	+				May be reduced		
Diuretics i Thiazides						May cause impotence	
ii Spironolactone				? blocks androgen receptors	Maybe reduced (can also cause gynaecomastia)	May cause impotence	

Drug			Mechanism	Effect on libido	Effect on erection / potency	Effect on ejaculation
Hormones						
i Androgens Testosterone	+		Peripheral effects on genitals	Females — increased, Males — increased (if androgen deficient)	May improve (if androgen-deficient)	May cause ejaculatory delay
ii Corticosteroids	+		Antagonize testosterone	Reduced	May cause impotence	
iii Oestrogens	+			Males reduced	May cause impotence. May increase response in females	Ejaculatory delay
Hypnotics Barbiturates	+			?Increased in low doses when anxiety present. Reduced with high doses.	? Increased in low doses when anxiety present. Impotence with high doses.	Delayed in high doses.
Major tranquillizers Phenothiazines Thioridazine	?	+		May be reduced	May cause eretile failure	Often causes retrograde ejaculation
Chlorpromazine	?	+		May be reduced	May cause erectile failure	
Opiates Morphine	+			Reduced	Impotence in high doses.	Inhibited in high doses.
Other drugs Disulfiram			Unknown	Decreased	Decreased	Delayed ejaculation
Tryptophan	+					
Ephedrine			Alpha-adrenergic stimulation			Rapid ejaculation

From Hawton, K. (1982). Sexual problems in the general hospital. In *Medicine and Psychiatry — A Practical Approach*, eds Creed, F.H. and Pfeffer, J.M. Pitman Publishing Ltd, London.

other hand is often associated with organic pathology, the site of which determines whether pain is felt immediately on intercourse or on deep penetration. Common causes of dyspareunia include

Superficial
local painful lesions
vaginismus

inadequate vaginal
lubrication

Deep
endometriosis
pelvic inflammatory
disease
ovarian cysts and tumours

Where there is no organic pathology then, as with penile pain, it is due to psychological factors; for example, vaginismus and inadequate vaginal lubrication may be due to lowered arousal.

SEXUAL DEVIATIONS (see Table 6.5)

Homosexuality

Though this is included in the table of sexual deviancies, the attitude towards it has become increasingly liberal in the last two decades. Homosexuality is defined as sexual thoughts, feelings or acts towards a member of the same sex. Both male and female homosexuality occur both exclusively and as part of a bisexual orientation.

Table 6.5 Sexual deviations

1 Abnormality of orientation	homosexuality, male and female
2 Abnormality of the sexual object	fetishism transvestism paedophilia bestiality necrophilia incest
3 Abnormality of the sexual act	exhibitionism voyeurism sadism masochism frotteurism rape
4 Abnormality of gender role	transsexualism gender disturbance in children

Adapted from Gelder, F.M., Gath, D. and Mayou, R. (1983). *Oxford Textbook of Psychiatry*. Oxford University Press.

It is especially prevalent in adolescents and in single-sex establishments, and population studies have suggested that ten per cent of males are more or less exclusively homosexual for at least three years and that four per cent of men and a similar percentage of women remain persistently homosexual. Aetiological factors include abnormal relationships with parents, sociocultural sexual mores and social and sexual anxieties.

Homosexuals show the same range of psychological disorders as do heterosexuals.

Abnormality of the sexual object

Fetishism is predominantly a male sexual deviation and is defined as the use of objects, such as clothing, as the usual way of evoking sexual arousal. *Transvestism*, found in both sexes, is dressing in clothing of the opposite sex and may be associated with transsexualism and homosexuality, although many patients are heterosexual. *Paedophilia* (see chapter 10) is sexual activity with prepubertal children in preference to adults. It occurs almost exclusively in men and the relationship may be a heterosexual or a homosexual one. Sexual arousal may also be achieved with animals in *bestiality* and with dead bodies in *necrophilia*.

Incest involves sexual activity between members of a nuclear family, particularly between fathers and daughters. Because of social and legal prohibitions it is volunteered infrequently though it is probably not uncommon.

Abnormality of the sexual act

Exhibitionism (indecent exposure) is the inappropriate display of genitalia and/or other sexual areas in order to achieve sexual gratification (see chapter 10). *Voyeurism* is the obtaining of arousal by watching others engaged in sexual behaviour or in states of undress and is also associated with masturbation either to the act or to the memory of it. *Sadism* is the practice of inflicting pain as part of sexual behaviour while in *masochism* arousal is obtained by being the object of sadistic or humiliating sexual behaviour. *Frotteurism* is the achievement of sexual excitement by rubbing against an unwilling partner often in a crowded place such as a train. Other abnormalities include the association of sexual excitement with either fantasies or observation of defecation, urination and vomiting.

In *rape*, intercourse, either heterosexual or homosexual, occurs against consent and may be accompanied by violence and murder (see chapter 10).

Abnormality of gender role

Transsexualism

Transsexuals are convinced that their sexual gender is different from that shown by the external genitalia and this is associated with a wish to change or correct the so-called anatomical disorder. In order to live their life according to their preferred sexual gender they usually cross-dress. It occurs most commonly in males but may also be present in females.

Transsexualism usually starts in childhood with a preference for pursuits and activities of members of the opposite, desired gender. However other children who also show behaviour, including dressing, which is out of keeping with their true sexual gender grow up with normal sexual habits.

Aetiological factors in sexual deviations (see Table 6.6)

Table 6.6 Aetiological factors in sexual deviation

Disturbed relationships with parents

Parental marital disharmony

Social and sexual anxieties and difficulties

Antisocial (psychopathic) personality disorders especially with associated violence

Aberrant conditioning where sexual attitudes and behaviour are wrongly learnt

Low IQ

Alcohol abuse

Mental illness — mania, dementia, obsessive compulsive neurosis

Genetic factors

Possibly prenatal endocrine factors

Disorder relating to sexuality

Disorders of menstruation

Premenstrual tension A number of research studies have shown that the time preceding and during menstruation tends to be a time when women are more likely to present with psychiatric problems. There is also an increase in aggressive behaviour, accidents, alteration in sexual arousal and behaviour and impaired performance on various psychological tests. The physical symptoms of premenstrual tension include painful tender breasts, a feeling of swelling, backache, headache, skin eruption and stomach cramps. The psychological symptoms include tension, irritability, depression, tiredness, sleep disturbance, mood swings, forgetfulness, and feelings of loneliness. There are also behavioural symptoms including clumsiness, proneness to accidents, a tendency to avoid social situations and loss of efficiency.

Premenstrual tension can start at any time after puberty but is more common in the thirties and forties, and is often associated with irregular, heavy or painful periods. Since the psychological and behavioural symptoms are nonspecific, controversy surrounds its existence as an entity, and in particular its discrimination from similar symptoms in women with pre-existing neuroses. The current evidence suggests that PMT is an exceedingly common complaint of neurotic women, but that it also, more rarely, is experienced by women with normal psychological adjustment. The most important diagnostic test is a diary, kept by the women for three months, which records her menstruation and all the physical and psychological abnormalities of which she complains. Many women will be surprised to find that mood swings, outbursts of temper etc occur throughout the cycle and are not related to menstruation; some display a definite cycle. Theories as to its aetiology include hormonal imbalance and women's attitudes to menstruation.

The Menopause The menopause is a time when women may complain of psychiatric symptoms though there is no body of research evidence to indicate that these are hormone-related. However the menopause is a time of change of role with the children growing up and leaving home with consequent pressure on the marital relationship. This would suggest that symptoms occurring at the menopause may be due to psychological reasons, and this is lent further support by the finding of similar psychological changes in men due to so-called mid-life crises.

Disorders of Pregnancy

During Pregnancy Minor psychological problems including depression and anxiety are not uncommon during pregnancy especially in the first trimester, and are related to psychological complaints before pregnancy. Sexual drive may also be altered with a reduction in drive in the last trimester and the first few months after birth. Excess vomiting in pregnancy — hyperemesis gravidarum — may also be related to psychological problems.

After Birth Most women have a brief period of depression and anxiety on the third or fourth day after parturition (the 'blues') which usually resolves in a couple of days without treatment and is related to hormonal changes. About ten per cent of women develop longer-lasting states of depression with onset usually in the first few weeks after pregnancy and associated with impairment of sleep, appetite and libido. These are probably due to psychological rather than hormonal factors and are caused by the difficulty of adjusting to a new role in life.

Finally a very small number of women — 1.5 per 1000 deliveries — will develop puerperal psychoses, usually in the first two weeks post partum. The symptomatology may be mixed although two-thirds are predominantly affective and one-third schizophrenic. Organic psychoses, for example due to gross anaemia or post partum infection, are now rare in countries with advanced obstetric care. However women with functional puerperal psychoses frequently show a degree of clouding of consciousness and disorientation and care must be taken that a diagnosis of organic aetiology is not missed.

The most significant predictors of post partum psychosis are a family and previous psychiatric history of psychotic illness. This tends to support the current majority view: that post partum psychosis is not a specific illness but part of a genetically determined susceptibility to functional psychosis and that the puerperium, in terms of both its physiological and its psychological stress, is a particularly likely precipitant of an attack. Some authors however argue that the phenomenology of post partum psychosis is so specific as to justify its discrimination as a separate illness.

Pseudocyesis Some women develop ideas that they are pregnant at a time when this is not the case. In certain situations this is related to the wish to have children and may be found in people with psychosexual personality problems. In some people this idea reaches delusional proportions — for example, when intercourse has not occurred for many years or may never have occurred. These patients may be depressed or schizophrenic or this may be an isolated delusion. In some patients it recurs depending on the underlying illness or the evironmental situation.

Couvade Some men develop symptoms during their partner's pregnancy which are commonly complained of by pregnant women. This is a rare, self-limiting disorder.

Abnormal self-image of genitalia

Some patients complain that their genitalia are abnormal but on physical examination there is no evidence of this. The complaints may also occur with other secondary sexual characteristics such as breasts, though this may be dictated by prevailing socal mores. Where the self-image is abnormal the symptom is called dysmorphophobia (see Chapter 2).

Koro is a rare disease in which men believe their penis to have shrunk inside their bodies. Though initially reported in the Far East cases have been described in the Western world. The underlying diagnosis may be schizophrenia or obsessive compulsive neurosis.

CASE HISTORY
JOHN BROWN

Mr John Brown, a 30-year-old unemployed man, went to his general practitioner with a one-to-two-year history of inability to maintain an erection during sexual intercourse with his wife. As a result of this the marriage was becoming increasingly fraught and his wife had threatened to leave with their eighteen-month-old adopted son unless he got his sexual problem sorted out. On further questioning it appeared that he still, at times, woke up in the morning with normal erections and was able to masturbate normally. He had gone to prostitutes to see if there would be any difference there but although he had succeeded on the first occasion he had failed on three subsequent ones. To make matters worse he felt guilty about these liaisons and was worried in case he had caught a venereal infection which he might pass on to his wife.

In his past medical history he had developed mumps at the age of 23 soon after his marriage and this had left him sterile. He had only found this out when, after trying unsuccessfully for a child for years, the couple had gone to the doctor for investigation of infertility. The only other point of relevance in the medical history was that there was a strong family history of diabetes though he had not been tested for this and there were no symptoms suggestive of diabetes or of any other major physical illness.

On discussing his marriage Mr Brown said that initially the couple had been happy together with a full enjoyable sex life and this was confirmed by his wife. His wife for her part desperately wanted a child and had cooled towards him when she found out he was infertile. She had insisted on adopting a child and he had somewhat reluctantly agreed to this. However their sex life had deteriorated since then and whereas this had not initially distressed her unduly, as she was up at nights with their infant son, over the last few months she become increasingly frustrated and was threatening to end their marriage. A further complicating factor was that soon after the adoption Mr Brown had without warning been made redundant from the job he had since leaving school, as a machine tool operator. He had received only a limited amount of redundancy money, much less than he thought he deserved given his years of service. In the last year and a half despite looking hard he had been unable to find employment commensurate with his skills and experience. This not surprisingly had placed a further strain on the marriage. To make matters worse Mr Brown had started drinking, something which he could ill afford.

In his background there was no family psychiatric history. Both his parents were still alive and happily married and he saw them regularly if infrequently. He had two married sisters with whom he was also on good terms. His childhood was nothing out of the ordinary, he did reasonably well at school where he was popular and truanted occasionally with his peers. He was very good at sport and was proud of the fact that he had been captain of both football and cricket. After leaving school he had gone to work as an apprentice machine tool operator and continued his interest in sport by joining the local boxing club where he was known as 'Mr Tough'.

As an adolescent he had had plenty of girl-friends and was sexually experienced. There had been no episodes of impotence or any other type of sexual dysfunction and he had had no homosexual tendencies or experiences. He met his wife at a dance when he was eighteen, they lived together soon after this and were married four years later. At interview Mr Brown seemed uneasy when talking about his sexual problem and there was some evidence of a mild but appropriate degree of unhappiness. There were no other abnormal findings in his mental state or physical examination.

Questions

What factors would lead you to think that Mr Brown's impotence was psychological rather than organic in nature?
What are the aetiological factors?
What is the prognosis?

The presence of erections on waking in the morning and on masturbation would not be consistent with an organic cause when one would expect the failure of arousal to be global and not situation-specific. In addition, as shown below, there are ample psychological causes to explain his impotence. Nevertheless, given the strong family history of diabetes it would be wise to rule this out despite the psychological picture, in case it was a contributory factor to what would still be largely psychologically caused impotence.

One important factor is the loss of self-esteem and manliness occasioned by finding out that he was sterile. This is supported by his reluctance to adopt a child and the previous importance given to being a 'man' — hence his sporting pursuits and his nickname 'Mr Tough'. These feelings would have been further enhanced by his redundancy in distressing circumstances and his inability to obtain alternative suitable employment. Impotence is often a sign of anger with a sexual partner, that is the withholding of sexual favours. This may to some extent be relevant to the Browns with Mr Brown being angry with his wife's insistence on adoption and also on his going to the doctor to display his loss of manliness. Further factors include his guilt and anxiety following his liaisons with prostitutes, his increased alcohol consumption and his general unhappiness with his present situation. Finally there is often an element of performance anxiety: failure on one occasion leads to anxiety on the next and thereby to further failure, as arousal is to a large extent controlled by higher cortical centres and anxiety is a powerful inhibitory factor.

The prognosis in secondary erectile impotence is usually very good with behavioural treatment. Treatment in this case would necessitate helping Mr Brown to come to terms with his sterility and redundancy, advising him to cut down his drinking, and dealing with his anxieties about any venereal infection he might have picked up, while helping the couple to resolve their marital stress; as well as a specific behavioural programme for his impotence.

7

Alcohol and drug abuse

Alcohol is probably the most widely used and abused psychotropic drug. It is estimated that there are three quarters of a million to one million people with drinking problems in this country, and 10 per cent of the population can be classed as heavy drinkers. This figure has increased rapidly over the last 25 years. It has been estimated that 65 per cent of home accidents are caused, in part at least, by alcohol; that 1 in 3 medical admissions, and 1 in 10 psychiatric admissions, are alcohol-related; and that in a high proportion of murders and road traffic accidents alcohol is involved. Finally there is $2\frac{1}{2}$ times as much absenteeism among problem drinkers as amongst the rest of the population.

TERMINOLOGY

The DHSS Advisory Committee on Alcoholism has proposed the term 'problem drinkers' for those who suffer alcohol-related disabilities from repeated drinking. It has been suggested that there are three groups of patients whose drinking behaviour may lead to problems: there are those who drink excessively, those who become intoxicated and those who suffer from alcohol dependence (see below). These groups may occur independently or in combination in the same individual.

MODELS

One of the problems in the management and prevention of alcohol-related disability is the divergence of conceptual models. Alcoholism may be seen, on the one hand, as an illness for which the patient is not responsible and from which he never truly recovers — once an alcoholic always an alcoholic. This, the view of Alcoholics Anonymous, places the responsibility for treatment firmly with society and is in marked contrast to a second model which is that alcoholism is deviant behaviour for which the patient is fully responsible. Both models have their fervent adherents and both have advantages and disadvantages. Because of this it is clinically most effective to treat each person as an individual without any rigid framework.

AETIOLOGICAL FACTORS

These include availability of alcohol; social and cultural drinking habits; occupation, for example those working in breweries, involved in business

Table 7.1 Aetiological factors in alcoholism

Family background	genetic
	environmental
Social & cultural	general level of alcohol consumption in the population or the patient's subgroup
	association of alcohol with occupation or social life
	ease of availability
Economic	relative cost of alcohol
Psychological Factors	as tranquillizer
	following traumatic life event including loss of role
	personality difficulties
Physical	to relieve withdrawal symptoms
	to ease pain

lunches, in the armed forces, merchant navy, etc; the individual's physical state and psychopathology including his personality and mood; precipitating life events, for example break-up of a marriage; and family background (see Table 7.1).

PHYSIOLOGICAL EFFECTS

Though alcohol may appear to be a stimulant, it is in fact a central nervous system depressant with effects on judgement, behavioural performance, motor skills and mood. The psychological signs and symptoms include merriment, querulousness, moroseness, disinhibition and violence. The exact nature and degree of effect depend on the dose of alcohol, the individual's metabolism, the environment in which it is drunk and the personality and prevailing mood of the drinker. Though in certain circumstances, for example in the presence of severe anxiety or difficulties in socializing, alcohol may have a beneficial effect, generally it produces both mental and physical impairment. Acute physical effects include ataxia, slurring of speech, nausea, vomiting and diuresis. Central nervous depression causes somnolence and lowered levels of consciousness though paradoxically sleep impairment may occur. Hangovers after a bout of drinking are common and there may be amnesia for the night before. When very excessive amounts of alcohol are drunk alcohol poisoning may occur, which can be fatal.

CLINICAL ASPECTS

Presentation

Some people present directly with drinking problems and others are presented by families or friends. However, many heavy drinkers first present via one of the alcohol-related disabilities (see Table 7.4). The presence therefore of any of these symptoms should alert one to the possibility of alcohol abuse. Additional factors which should lead to suspicion are a family history of alcoholism and a high risk occupation. Even where these do not exist a drinking history should be taken from all patients.

History

A detailed drinking history involves asking about a representative drinking day, enquiring into the pattern of drinking, amount and duration of drinking, and any precipitating factors and ensuing problems, including withdrawal symptoms. An independent informant may give a more reliable account than the patient himself.

Patterns of drinking

People may drink socially or excessively or may be abstinent. Excessive drinking may occur in bouts (benders) or may be continuous. Bouts may be precipitated by stress or may depend on the financial situation of the patient. In the alcohol dependence syndrome, drinking occurs to relieve withdrawal symptoms and the drinking repertoire is narrowed. Drinking may occur at home or in public, alone or in company. It is difficult to give a figure for excessive alcohol consumption as this must to some extent vary from person to person. However if one takes the risk of developing cirrhosis as the level of excessive alcohol consumption then for men this is about a daily consumption of 80 ml (8 units) of absolute alcohol (4 pints of beer or its equivalent; see Table 7.2), while for women it is at the much lower level of 30 ml of absolute alcohol daily. At a level of 8 pints of beer daily there is a great risk of developing alcohol dependence.

Table 7.2 Units of alcohol

1 unit of alcohol	= one half pint of beer
	= one single spirit
	= one glass of sherry
	= one glass of wine

One bottle of spirits	= 30 units
One bottle of table wine	= 7 units
One bottle of sherry	= 12 units

Adapted from Thorley, A. Medical responses to problem drinking. *Medicine Series No. 3*, **35**, 1816–1822.

Laboratory investigations

Blood alcohol levels should be estimated in all patients in whom heavy drinking is suspected. A high blood alcohol level without corresponding effects on the patient's behaviour suggests tolerance. One disadvantage of this investigation is that blood alcohol is subject to rapid decay. Other abnormal findings which alert one to heavy drinking are a raised Mean Corpuscular Volume (MCV) without adequate explanation (found in 40% of dependent individuals) and abnormal liver function tests especially gamma glutamyl transpeptidase (γ GT) raised in 70–80% of dependent drinkers as well as in some heavy social drinkers. The heavier the consumption, the higher the γ GT, which does not come back to normal until about eleven days after stopping drinking. γ GT is also increased by enzyme-inducing drugs such as phenytoin and barbiturates and by liver disease, pancreatitis and myocardial infarction. AST (SGOT) and SGPT (serum glutamic pyruvic transaminase) are often raised in the middle of a heavy drinking bout while remaining normal in steady drinking. GDH (glutamate dehydrogenase) is a good indicator of active alcohol liver disease while alpha-amino-n-butyric acid/leucine ratio and

Table 7.3 Short Michigan alcoholism screening test (Mast)

1 Do you feel you are a normal drinker? (by normal we mean you drink less than or as much as most other people)

2 Does your wife, husband, a parent, or other near relative ever worry or complain about your drinking?

3 Do you ever feel guilty about your drinking?

4 Do friends or relatives think you are a normal drinker?

5 Are you able to stop drinking when you want to?

6 Have you ever attended a meeting of Alcoholics Anonymous?

7 Has drinking ever created problems between you and your wife, husband, a parent or other near relative?

8 Have you ever got into trouble at work because of drinking?

9 Have you ever neglected your obligations, your family, or your work for two or more days in a row because you were drinking?

10 Have you ever gone to anyone for help about your drinking?

11 Have you ever been in hospital because of drinking?

12 Have you ever been arrested for drunken driving, driving while intoxicated, or driving under the influence of alcoholic beverages?

13 Have you ever been arrested, even for a few hours, because of other drunken behaviour?

Murray, R.M. and Bernadt, M. Early detection of alcoholism. *Medicine Series No. 3*, 35, 1811–1815.

Table 7.4 Cage questionnaire

1 Have you ever felt you ought to cut down on your drinking?

2 Have people annoyed you by criticizing your drinking?

3 Have you ever felt bad or guilty about your drinking?

4 Have you ever had a drink first thing in the morning to steady your nerves or get rid of a hangover ('eye-opener')?

Robin M, Murray and Morris Bernadt: Early detection of alcoholism, *Medicine Series No. 3*, 35, 1816–1822

serum transferrin are useful in detection of heavy drinkers but are not usually easily available in laboratories.

Questionnaires

These can be used as a screening tool. One of the best is the Michigan (see Table 7.3) a shortened version of which is the CAGE Questionnaire (see Table 7.4).

ALCOHOL DEPENDENCE SYNDROME

The alcohol dependence syndrome is characterized by the following points:

1 Withdrawal symptoms occur within 8–12 hours after abstinence. These include tremor, nausea, sweating and mood disturbance.

2 Relief is obtained by drinking more alcohol.

3 Drinking therefore becomes the behaviour most important to the sufferer.

4 As drinking occurs to relieve or avoid withdrawal symptoms the drinking pattern becomes narrowed when compared with that of the non-dependent drinker whose consumption varies from day to day.

5 Drinking becomes uncontrollable so that once started it is difficult to stop.

6 Drinking after a period of abstinence leads to a resurgence of the alcohol dependence syndrome.

7 Tolerance develops as indicated by very high blood levels of alcohol with little evidence of intoxication.

INTOXICATION

Most people can consume a particular amount of alcohol; alcohol consumed above this level causes intoxication. Problems related to intoxication are categorized in Table 7.5. However some individuals develop a phenomenon called pathological drunkenness after relatively small amounts of alcohol, probably as the result of an idiosyncratic reaction. These episodes are characterized by aggressive outbursts, with features of psychosis but no neurological signs of intoxication (see Chapter 16).

ALCOHOL-RELATED DISABILITIES

These may be psychological, physical or social (see Table 7.5).

Table 7.5 Problems related to elements of drinking behaviour

Physical and psychiatric problems

Intoxication

acute alcohol poisoning	acute gastritis	acute hypoglycaemia
acute myopathy	acute pancreatitis	amnesia
drug overdose	epilepsy	hangover
head injury	parasuicide	peripheral nerve pressure palsies

Chronic excessive intake

alcoholic hepatitis	alcoholic amblyopia	alcoholic ketoacidosis
carcinoma of mouth, pharynx, larynx or oesophagus	cardiomyopathy	central pontine myelinolyis
	fatty liver	cirrhosis
chronic cerebellar syndrome	chronic myopathy	dementia
cognitive dysfunction	Cushingoid syndrome	feminization
diabetes mellitus	epilepsy	gastrointestinal haemorrhage
fetal alcohol syndrome	gastritis	hyperlipidaemia
haemochromatosis	hepatoma	macrocytic anaemia
hyperuricaemia	impotence	oesophageal varices
malabsorption syndrome	Marchiafava-Bignami syndrome	pneumonia
peptic ulcer		suicide
reactive hypoglycaemia	peripheral neuropathy	Wernicke-Korsakov syndrome
tuberculosis	recurrent pancreatitis	
	vitamin deficiency	

Dependence

anxiety	delirium tremens	depression
epilepsy	hallucinations	paranoid states
phobias		

Social problems

Intoxication

absenteeism	child abuse	child neglect
domestic accidents	domestic violence	inappropriate aggression
inappropriate passivity	industrial accidents	sexual problems
social isolation		

Chronic excessive intake

debt	employment problems	family problems
homelessness	sexual problems	

Legal problems

Intoxication

assault	criminal damage	driving offences
drunk and disorderly	drunk and incapable	homicide
theft		

Chronic excessive intake

theft	vagrancy	violent behaviour including homicide

Adapted from Thorley, A. Medical Responses to Problem Drinking. *Medicine Series No. 3*, **35**, 1816–1822

Psychological

Acute organic brain disease (acute confusional state)

a Delirium tremens

In the presence of the alcohol dependence syndrome, withdrawal symptoms such as tremor, anxiety, nausea and sweating occur within 8–12 hours of abstinence. This may be followed by visual hallucinations during the first day, fits on the second and within a further twenty-four hours a full-blown confusional state with abnormal perceptions and autonomic overactivity. Delirium tremens usually remits in 1–3 days but may last for over a week. Restlessness, ataxia, frightening visual hallucinations and illusions, paranoid delusions and a mood characterized by extreme terror make up the clinical picture. Untreated it carries a significant risk of mortality due to suicide, intercurrent infection and circulatory collapse.

b Wernicke's encephalopathy and Korsakov's psychosis

These are caused by thiamine deficiency, which in the problem drinker is due to poor dietary intake. Wernicke's encephalopathy presents as an acute confusional state associated with opthalmoplegia, nystagmus and ataxia. The symptoms improve with thiamine, the neurological symptoms first while the confusional state usually lasts over a week (as compared to delirium tremens). If it is untreated or inadequately treated then a Korsakov's psychosis may result with an inability to learn new memories leading to confabulation (see Chapter 19). The prognosis for resolution is poor even with thiamine replacement unless this is achieved early in the illness.

Chronic brain disease

Alcohol-induced dementia

With the advent of the CAT scan and sophisticated psychological testing it has become increasingly apparent that a dementing process may occur as a result of excessive alcohol intake. The CAT scan shows generalized cortical atrophy and ventricular enlargement. Abstinence may be followed by a significant degree of improvement in intellectual function.

Functional psychoses

a Alcoholic hallucinosis

This is characterized by the presence of persecutory auditory hallucinations associated with anxiety, occurring in clear consciousness (see Chapter 18).

b Alcohol-induced paranoid psychoses

In this cases paranoid delusions dominate the picture. One example is the syndrome of morbid jealousy (see Chapters 9 and 17).

Mood Disturbance

Depression

Depression may be both a cause and an effect of problem drinking and may also occur after the patient has given up drinking. Overdoses are particularly common in heavy drinkers. Forty-five per cent of male and 16% of female patients who take overdoses are alcohol abusers. Alcohol increases the usual risk factors for suicide — namely physical and psychiatric ill-health, unemployment and social isolation — and its disinhibiting effect makes impulsive behaviour more likely.

Anxiety

Anxiety, similarly, may be a cause and an effect of problem drinking and is also the primary affect in acute withdrawal states. Phobias in particular may lead to heavy drinking as may social anxieties where alcohol is taken as 'Dutch courage'.

Personality Disorder

Many, but by no means all, patients who abuse alcohol have abnormal premorbid personalities. In addition heavy drinking with its organic, psychological and social sequelae takes its toll of the patient's personality.

Psychosexual Dysfunction

Drinking may lead to difficulties in erection and ejaculation as well as marital disharmony with secondary sexual difficulties.

Physical

Alcohol has long been known to produce cirrhosis but may also lead to damage in most of the other systems, especially neurological, gastrointestinal and cardiac (see Table 7.4).

Social

The picture of the alcoholic who starts adult life with a wife, family and job but who drifts downwards, loses his job, breaks with his family and passes from house to hostel to pavement is well-known. In addition, criminal offences may occur, either directly related to alcohol as are drink-driving offences, drunk and disorderly charges and violence; or as theft to finance drinking; or as sequelae of alcohol-induced psychological problems, for example, morbid jealousy.

DRUG DEPENDENCE

This is an increasing problem whether one considers opiate dependency, which is reaching epidemic proportions, or the use of minor tranquillizers such as diazepam. Solvent abuse in young children is a particularly topical problem.

Aetiological factors for drug abuse include personality disorders, subcultural pressures, social mores, emotional distress and physical illness where opiates are originally prescribed for pain relief. Many patients are polydrug and alcohol abusers. Sequelae are physical, including death from drug overdoses; psychological, for example, drug-induced psychoses; social; and forensic. Continued drug abuse may lead to both psychological and physical dependence. The symptoms produced on taking the drug and after its withdrawal differ according to the substance abused (see below). However, many of the drugs can cause acute psychoses and this must always be borne in mind when a patient is admitted with such a mental state.

Diagnosis of drug dependence

Three broad categories of drug misusers are recognized.
1 Stable drug misusers who do not experiment or substantially increase their dose and who have usually become dependent on drugs prescribed initially for physical illness. Chronic abuse of hypnotics and minor tranquillizers also comes into this category. However, due to their widespread availability, both from legal and black market sources, these drugs are popular with the more pathological polydrug abusers in groups *2* and *3*.
2 Young adults or adolescents who experiment with a variety of drugs, in varying doses, intermittently and depending on their social group, their finances and the availability of drugs. Most solvent abusers, amphetamine and LSD users are in this category. This group of abusers is at great risk of entering the third group.
3 Physically and psychologically dependent individuals, who consume drugs each day to the detriment of other activity. Their lives are centred around the procurement and use of drugs, they are frequently dependent on opiates and on barbiturates, and they are at greatest risk of conflict with the law, physical illness and death.

It is the increase in the second and third groups which is currently causing much concern in the UK, particularly because an increase in the experimenting group inevitably leads to an increase in the numbers of abnormally dependent abusers.

Drug abusers present to doctors in various ways. Some may frankly admit to a problem and seek help to withdraw from their drugs. Some may request a prescription of drugs, controlled or otherwise, without admitting to dependence, and others will complain of physical pain requiring analgesia. Many drug abusers claim to be dependent on larger doses than they in fact are, so that they can sell the excess; and a few dealers in drugs obtain them by claiming a dependence when they do not take drugs at all. The newly registered or newly referred patient is the most likely to attempt to obtain drugs by deceit.

Patients may also present via a physical complication such as septicaemia, abscess or hepatitis and may also develop an intercurrent illness such as appendicitis, when abrupt withdrawal may lead to complications in the clinical picture.

Physical examination

Drugs abusers who inject will have marks over veins in the arms, legs, groin or neck, and may have skin abscesses or thrombophlebitis. However many abusers do not inject but smoke, sniff or swallow drugs and there may be little evidence on physical examination. Polydrug users who abuse opiates may not show the characteristic pinpoint pupils of opiate addicts.

Investigations

Urine should be tested for types and amounts of drugs. Blood tests to check hepatitis B antigen and antibody status may be useful for future management.

Opiates

Effects	pleasure, warmth, tingling and relaxation.
Withdrawal	this occurs six hours after the last dose and peaks at 36–48 hours with symptoms of restlessness, insomnia, abdominal cramps, muscle and joint pains, runny eyes and nose, sweating, diarrhoea and vomiting, pilo-erection, dilated pupils, increased pulse rate and disturbance of temperature control.
Complications	reduced appetite and libido, constipation.
	central nervous system and respiratory depression which may be fatal.
	injection may lead to abscesses, septicaemia and hepatitis B.

Barbiturates

Effects	sedation, relaxation
Withdrawal	may produce a clinical syndrome comparable to delirium tremens. Epileptic fits are particularly common.
Complications	incoherence, slurred speech, nystagmus
	from injection as with opiates.
	death from overdose is common due to the relative toxicity of this drug.

Amphetamines

Effects	euphoria and stimulation, over-activity, wakefulness and anorexia sympathomimetic effects
Withdrawal	psychological not physical dependence, depression
Complications	cardiovascular complications may occur; malnutrition may result from anorexia.
	a paranoid psychosis indistinguishable from schizophrenia may occur with high doses and chronic abuse; a state resembling mania may also occur with large doses or in susceptible individuals.

Cocaine

Effects	stimulant: excitation as with amphetamines.
Withdrawal	psychological not physical dependence.
Complications	paranoid psychosis; formication: a feeling as of insects crawling under the skin.
	fits and dizziness, confusion and depression.
	perforation of nasal septum.

Hallucinogens

LSD

Effects	abnormal sensory perception, altered mood, including happiness and anxiety, bizarre behaviour.
	sympathomimetic effects
Withdrawal	nil
Complications	injury following bizarre behaviour, e.g. attempting to fly by jumping out of windows.
	flashback: recurrence of a 'trip' which may occur long after the drug was last taken
	paranoid psychoses may occur with auditory hallucinations, anxiety and restlessness, lasting from days to a few months.

Cannabis

Effects	increased feeling of wellbeing, altered perception.
Withdrawal	nil
Complications	acute paranoid psychosis and manic states. apathy with chronic abuse. conjunctival inflammation.

Solvent Abuse

Effects	initially excitation, euphoria and exhilaration followed by auditory or visual hallucinations and cerebral depressant effects.
Withdrawal	physical symptoms are rare but psychological dependence may occur.
Complications	neurological, encephalopathic, gastrointestinal symptoms: for example, abdominal pain, nausea and vomiting. death may occur following cerebral depression, asphyxia due to the plastic bag used in solvent inhalation, or inhalation of vomit.

Benzodiazepines

Effects	sedation, hypnosis
Withdrawal	physical dependence may lead to confusional states and convulsions. Psychological dependence causes rebound anxiety and insomnia. where benzodiazepines have been prescribed for anxiety withdrawal may be followed by recurrence of the initial condition.
Complications	impairment of judgment, disinhibition.

CASE HISTORY

MRS SWEENEY

Mrs Josephine Sweeney, a 48-year-old housewife, was referred by her general practitioner with a two-year history of increasing difficulty in coping at home. She was depressed and tearful and had at times felt that life was not worth living. She was arguing frequently with her husband and there was little sexual contact between them. Though he had a good job as a publican she was unable to manage on the money he gave her. She was late paying bills and had been threatened with having her electricity cut off. When helping her husband, serving behind the bar, she became irritable with customers and of late forgetful of their orders. She was sleeping poorly and eating very little but denied drinking except on social occasions.

She came from an Irish family who had settled in England when she was in her teens. Both her mother and father drank heavily and there were frequent arguments and fights at home. However, heavy drinking was the norm in the village where she was born. Her parents had died in their sixties, her father ten years ago of a perforated duodenal ulcer and her mother four years later from carcinoma of the breast. She was one of six children only one of whom was happily married. She had little contact with her siblings. Apart from heavy drinking there was no family psychiatric history.

Despite the arguments at home her childhood had not been too unhappy. On moving to England she had missed the friends she had left behind and, not being gregarious, she had difficulty making new ones. She met her husband when she was eighteen and married two years later. She had three children all of whom had left home within the last five years. There had been minor marital problems prior to this. Her only work outside the home after her marriage was helping her husband occasionally to run the pub, and she had no hobbies. However, prior to the children leaving home she had coped well. Her premorbid personality was that of a rather dependent and lonely woman.

Primary examination revealed a miserable middle-aged woman who looked older than her years and smelt of alcohol. She admitted being depressed but there was no evidence of paranoid delusions or auditory hallucinations. Brief testing of her cognitive state showed some memory impairment. Physical examination revealed spider naevi on her face and upper trunk, an enlarged liver and erythematous palms. There were no neurological abnormalities.

Her husband when interviewed on his own said that though she had always been a social drinker she had been drinking much more heavily recently. In the mornings her hands would shake and she was often sick. The housework had been neglected and she made many mistakes when serving behind the bar, to an extent that was now affecting his trade.

Questions

What hints in her history should alert one to the diagnosis of alcohol abuse and how could this be confirmed?

What are the aetiological factors?

What alcohol-induced physical and psychological sequelae does Mrs Sweeney appear to be developing?

There is the family history of heavy drinking, her background in Ireland where heavy drinking was accepted, her marital disharmony, inability to cope financially, increasing forgetfulness and the ready availability of alcohol whilst serving behind the bar. The abnormalities on physical examination are indicative of liver damage, which is commonly due to alcoholism, and this diagnosis is further supported by the fact that she smells of alcohol. Finally her husband's account shows that she is drinking to the extent of developing withdrawal symptoms in the morning.

Confirmatory evidence could be obtained by doing a blood alcohol level, an MCV looking for macrocytosis and a gamma GT and other liver function tests. The patient's denial of heavy drinking is not unusual and a full detailed drinking history should be taken (see text). Finally the presence of withdrawal symptoms on cessation of drinking following admission to hospital would confirm the diagnosis. This is a risky procedure and necessitates careful monitoring.

The long term aetiological factors include a possible genetic role, in that both parents were heavy drinkers, as well as an environmental one, since during her childhood she would have been exposed to a milieu in which heavy drinking was commonplace and acceptable. As for mid-term factors it is interesting to speculate on the role of her depression and marital disharmony in the genesis of her alcoholism. Her childhood view of marriage would have been conditioned by what she saw at home and might have predisposed her to the development of marital problems in later life. Most of the rest of her siblings had poor experience of marriage. This together with her dependence and difficulty in making friends may have resulted in an overdependence on her children which to some extent had mitigated the effects of her marital problems. However when they left home she was thrown more and more into the sole company of her husband at a time when she was already suffering from a marked loss of role. This probably led to her depression and drinking both of which would have increased her social isolation and thereby worsened her depression. This together with her increasing irritability would have had a further deleterious effect on the marital situation. Thus a vicious circle would have been set up leading to increasing alcohol abuse. This would have been further helped by the ready availability of alcohol in the pub where she and her husband work. Finally there is evidence of physical dependence on alcohol, providing a further more immediate precipitating factor to her increased drinking.

As mentioned above there is evidence of withdrawal symptoms first thing in the morning suggesting a degree of physical dependence on alcohol. A physical examination shows evidence of liver damage which should be confirmed by further investigations. Her cognitive impairment may be related to her depressed mood or may mark the onset of an alcohol-induced dementia. Psychometric studies and a CAT scan may help to clarify this though the former may need to be conducted serially. Her poor diet may predispose her towards developing a Wernicke-Korsakov syndrome and this must be borne in mind. Finally as regards her depression, though this may be an aetiological factor in her drinking it may also be a sequel of it. The links between depression and alcoholism are often very complex and difficult to tease out.

8

Failure to cope/nervous breakdown

Although doctors in general, and psychiatrists in particular, tend to focus primarily on symptoms and signs in the mental state which denote psychiatric illness, the major preoccupation of the patient which governs whether and when he presents for help is the degree to which the emotional disturbance intrudes into his everyday life and affects his ability to cope. Thus few patients will complain directly, for example, of hearing voices but many will say, 'Doctor I just can't cope any more,' or will be presented by relatives or friends as not coping. When this inability to cope becomes very severe, leading to time off work or withdrawal to bed, then this may be described by the term nervous breakdown (though this has in addition connotations of overtly bizarre behaviour). Nervous breakdown is a lay term which covers a multitude of different psychiatric diagnoses, all of which have as their common denominator the effect of affecting the ability to cope.

Failure to cope may be situation-specific, as with the housewife who is unable to do her housework but functions normally at bingo, or the businessman who cannot keep up at work but retains the capacity to be involved in his outside activities; or it may be a generalized inability to function at any level. The two may reflect very different psychiatric states, with the latter usually suggesting a more severe disorder

'Hysterics'

To the lay mind the concept of nervous breakdown usually implies an outburst of uncontrolled behaviour such as screaming, shouting and shaking. This behaviour is often referred to as hysterical; but should not be confused with the technical use of this term in psychiatry to denote hysterical neuroses. Dramatic, histrionic behaviour *per se* indicates no particular diagnosis other than distress, and/or demand for attention. It may be more frequent in patients with hysterical personality disorders as they lurch from crisis to crisis, but may also occur in people without psychiatric disorder or in those who are anxious and depressed. It should not be confused with the catastrophic reaction of anger or dismay experienced by those suffering from dementia.

GENERALIZED INABILITY TO COPE (see Table 8.1)

Mood disorder

A disturbance of mood is probably the commonest psychological reason for a generalized inability to cope. Depression may lead to loss of energy, sleep impairment with subsequent tiredness, decreased appetite and weight causing weakness, loss of interest in self and surroundings, loss of self-

Table 8.1 Generalized inability to cope

Mood disorder
Lack of energy
Lack of drive
Low self-esteem and self-confidence
Impairment of intellect
Physical illness with psychological overlay
Personality disorders
Self-inflicted inability to cope
Preoccupation with other matters
Obsessive compulsive neuroses

esteem and self-confidence, impairment of concentration and pseudodementia, motor agitation or retardation, all of which will impair the ability and/or desire to carry out normal daily functions. Similarly, the anxious patient may complain of fatigue, subsequent to both sleep impairment and the increased level of arousal; powers of attention and concentration may be reduced as may be the ability to tolerate frustration. Though the manic patient may be so involved in other activities as to neglect home and work *he* is unlikely to complain of an inability to cope, rather believing that his ability to cope is increased; but his relatives or friends or employers will be more perturbed about the effects on his daily life.

Lack of energy

This may be secondary to depression or anxiety, to sedative drugs or alcohol, to physical illness or to sleep impairment. The ICD–9 includes the term neurasthenia (300.5) for a neurotic disorder characterized by 'fatigue, irritability, headache, depression, insomnia, difficulty in concentration and lack of capacity for enjoyment'. This was at one time a fashionable diagnosis and included concepts such as nervous exhaustion due to overwork. However despite its continued presence in the ICD–9 it is likely that although the symptom constellation certainly exists, it is not a distinct entity, but part of an associated neurotic depression, anxiety neurosis or hysterical disorder. Post-traumatic neuroses may present a similar clinical picture. Patients with anorexia nervosa commonly indulge in excessive exercise but if their food intake is low enough they may complain of lethargy as well as a physical inability to cope. Finally patients from some cultures, for example those from the Indian subcontinent, with emotional disorders, may present primarily with a feeling of lethargy or weakness often accompanied by physical symptoms.

Lack of drive

Apathy or lack of volition is one of the classical symptoms of schizophrenia especially when the disease is chronic. However the patient, although manifestly not coping, is unlikely to complain of this. Demented and depressed patients may also suffer from lack of drive and this may be shown by their lack of personal hygiene and self-neglect. Lack of self care is further discussed in Chapter 2.

Low self-esteem and self-confidence

This may be a symptom of depression, anxiety, of personality disorder — inadequate and dependent in type — or of post-traumatic neurosis. Chronic unemployment is also likely to lead to low self-esteem and self-confidence and may result in the person being unable to cope in any sphere.

Impairment of intellect

The ability to cope with tasks is to a large extent dependent on a person's intellectual capacity. This may always have been low as in mental retardation; or it may have become impaired either by an organic process such as dementia (or a confusional state), or by a functional disorder affecting the ability to think (e.g. schizophrenia) or to concentrate (depression and anxiety). In the more gross forms of intellectual impairment, the patient commonly lacks insight into his disability and it is the relatives or friends who will ask for help, as in the instance of the demented wife brought up by her husband with the complaint that she is continually leaving gas taps on. However in the early stages of dementia the patient may be aware of his difficulties and may present because of them. In these cases the situation is further adversely affected when the insightful patient becomes depressed about his failing intellectual powers.

Physical illness with psychological overlay

Obviously severe physical illness will greatly impair the ability to cope with everyday tasks but this is outside the scope and remit of this book. However, even when true physical pathology exists, there is sometimes a large subjective component. It has been suggested that in chronic bronchitis, a severe disabling disorder, breathlessness which limits activity may in some cases be determined more by attitudes and beliefs than by lung pathology. Similarly with rheumatoid arthritis, many patients will be able to come to terms with their handicap while others may exaggerate the symptoms because of personality or emotional problems.

Personality disorders

An individual's personality will to a large extent determine how he copes with adversity and whether he denies or exaggerates his disabilities. Thus some patients will deny their problems and resume work within days of surgery, while others will convalesce for months after the same operation, insisting that they are not well enough to cope with normal activities. Some people may set themselves such high standards that anything less than 100% is viewed as failure, whereas others are happy living in surroundings which would suggest to the onlooker that they were neglecting themselves. On the other hand the professed inability to cope may be objectively untrue, but may be presented in order to manipulate circumstances either as a way of managing intolerable stress or for financial or other gain.

Self-inflicted inability to cope

Alcohol and drug abuse may lead to an inability to carry out normal tasks whether due to intoxication or to secondary psychiatric illness. Dependence on psychotropic drugs may lead the person to feel he is unable to cope without them while at the same time causing sedation, psychomotor impairment and disinhibition. Both anorexia nervosa and obesity may lead to physical sequelae which render the patient so unfit as grossly to impair any normal activity.

Preoccupation with other matters

Life crisis

Major life crises may so preoccupy the patient that every waking minute is spent thinking about the matter in hand to the detriment of everyday tasks. Secondary anxiety and/or depression may also take its toll, or the patient may cope with stress by developing an hysterical conversion or dissociative state or a psychogenic psychosis, during which normal function is either lost or severely impaired. One major life crisis which usually upsets the normal routine is a bereavement, and this will be dealt with in more detail.

Grief reaction

Loss, whether by death or separation (for example, the breakup of a relationship) is usually followed by the process of grieving. The exact nature of this is dependent on a number of factors including the sociocultural environment to which the patient belongs, his relationship with the lost object, his personality and past experiences, his current situation and the nature of the loss itself.

Though the particulars may differ, grieving usually follows a similar course starting with a period of denial followed by disturbance of mood with depression, tearfulness, sleep and appetite impairment, poor concentration, searching behaviour and symptoms of anxiety, and terminating in a phase of acceptance. During the second stage there may be ideas of guilt concerning lack of care for the deceased and/or hostility towards those who had looked after him. The bereaved may also experience the sensation of the presence of the deceased and undergo hallucinations relating to him. Physical symptoms are common and often suggest the illness from which the deceased died. Where the loss is due to the break-up of a relationship there may be suicidal and/or homicidal ideation and actions. The whole process usually lasts several months with the person being unable to carry out his normal activities for a period of some weeks.

In certain cases the grieving process is abnormal; either the grief is delayed or repressed, which may lead to the later development of psychiatric illnesses — depression and psychosomatic illness — or the grief may become prolonged or chronic. In the latter instance the patient is unable to stop grieving and cannot pick up the strings of life. Even where the grieving has been successfully coped with there may be exacerbations at the times of the anniversary of the loss or of significant events connected with the lost loved one or on the occasion of subsequent losses.

Obsessive-compulsive disorders

These have been defined as a recurrent or persistent thought, image, feeling, impulse or movement which is accompanied by an immediate sense of subjective compulsion and a desire to resist it, the event being recognized by the sufferer as foreign to his personality and into the nature of which he has insight. The ICD–9 definition of obsessive-compulsive disorders (300.3) is as follows:

> States in which the outstanding symptom is a feeling of subjective compulsion — which must be resisted — to carry out some action, to dwell on an idea, to recall an experience, or to ruminate on an abstract topic. Unwanted thoughts which intrude, the insistency of words or ideas, ruminations or trains of thought are perceived by the patient to be inappropriate or nonsensical. The obsessional urge or idea is recognized as alien to the personality but as coming from within the self. Obsessional actions may be quasi-ritual performances designed to relieve anxiety, e.g. washing the hands to cope with contamination. Attempts to dispel the unwelcome thoughts or urges may lead to a severe inner struggle, with intense anxiety.

Common compulsive rituals include cleaning — handwashing, bathing and house-cleaning based on fears of contamination; checking, based on obsessional doubts; dressing; tidying and counting, i.e. having to do an act a certain number of times. There is an element of obsessional doubting in many compulsive rituals which leads to them having to be repeated over and over again. Obsessional rituals may be so widespread and time-consuming as to leave no space for any other activities. On the other hand they may be specific to one sphere of life or even to one place. An example of the latter is the woman who makes everyone take off their shoes before entering the house in case they have been contaminated by outside objects. This then generalizes to insisting on members of the family taking a bath on coming home. The patient is still able to visit other people's houses without rituals but the conditions which she places on visitors have inevitably led to the reduction of her social activities.

By their very nature obsessional rituals prolong the time it would normally take for any activity and this may lead to lateness at work or social engagements or to a major curtailment of sleep. In certain situations obsessional slowness is the only feature and when it occurs in the absence of rituals or ruminations it is termed primary obsessional slowness.

Obsessive compulsive neurosis may be associated with depression; the obsession may be part of a depressive illness, or the depression may be secondary to the distress caused by the obsessional symptoms. In either case depression itself may have a further effect on the ability to cope. Finally some people are obsessionally tidy, houseproud or careful at work as part of their personality without having an obsessive compulsive neurosis as such, and this may lead to difficulties in coping both at home and at work.

SITUATIONAL COPING DIFFICULTIES (see Table 8.2)

Difficulties at home

Problems with coping primarily at home while being able to carry out external activities are due to relationship difficulties with those living at home, behaviour specifically linked to home, or environmental problems including inadequate housing.

Table 8.2 Situational coping difficulties

Difficulties at home
Relationship difficulties
   spouse or cohabitee
   children
   others at home

Behavioural problems specific to the home

Environmental difficulties

Difficulties at work
The job itself

The person doing the job

Relationships at work

Employment behaviour

Social Difficulties

Relationship difficulties

With spouse or cohabitee

Whereas in previous generations couples would usually have stayed together even when they were not content with each other, in recent years divorce and separation have become increasingly common. Psychiatric factors which may lead to marital disharmony include psychosexual and other personality difficulties and chronic psychiatric illness. Paradoxically, however, in phobic anxiety states the marriage may deteriorate when the disorder is successfully treated. This may be because the basis on which the relationship was founded was one of dependence. Women with anorexia nervosa are particularly likely to have unstable marriages, and obsessive compulsive neuroses may lead to intolerable domestic stress because of the coerced involvement of the whole family. Morbid jealousy or the abuse of alcohol or drugs by either partner is invariably associated with a poor marital relationship.

The sequelae of marital/couple disharmony include domestic violence (see Chapter 9) mood impairment of either party, sexual dysfunction and a severely strained atmosphere at home leading to home-based coping problems. An example of situation-specific difficulties is the patient, at loggerheads with her husband, who is well at work but develops severe tension headaches on the way home and at weekends.

With children

People who have never experienced adequate parenting themselves may have difficulties when they acquire this role as may those with personality difficulties in the areas of sexuality and dependence. This may lead to neglect, abuse (see Chapter 9) or overprotection, with subsequent psychological problems in the children which further aggravate the parents. On the other hand the children may themselves be difficult and young children may cause interruption of sleep, interfere with the privacy of their parents and lead to one, usually the female, becoming housebound. All this may cause maternal depression and resentment, with difficulties in coping at home and marital disharmony. This is particularly likely when there are a number of young children at home and when there is little support for the mother. For the obsessionally houseproud mother a little baby may present a severe challenge to her regime; while some fathers may see the children as rivals for the affections of their wife. Mothers with puerperal psychoses or post-partum depression are especially likely to be unable to cope with their family responsibilities.

With others at home

People living with parents may find themselves in a conflict of loyalties. This is especially so if the parent is elderly and infirm and needs looking after at the expense of the spouse or children. Lodgers or pets may also create problems.

Behavioural problems specific to the house

These consist largely of obsessional behaviour with rituals of house-cleaning. This may also be the case where one partner, though not suffering from an obsessive compulsive neurosis, is obsessionally houseproud while the other one is not.

Environmental problems

Housing which is inadequate either in its structure or in its social environment is understandably likely to lead to difficulties largely confined to the house, with an improvement in mental health in other situations. Specific problems may exist where the house has belonged to the partner's spouse from a previous marriage or where it is a constant reminder of a bereavement which occurred in that setting. Paranoid delusions may be solely directed to the home environment.

Difficulties at work.

Difficulty in coping at work may be due to factors within the job itself, changes in the person doing the job, relationships at work and general employment difficulties.

The job itself

Variables in the job include the amount of work,

the responsibility it entails, the nature of the job and the security of employment. There may be excessive amounts of work to be done to meet financial pressures, due to the obsessional personality of the person doing the job, or because the amount of work per person is unusually high. There may be increased responsibility with promotion at work and it is not unusual for someone who has coped well for many years suddenly to fail to cope soon after getting promotion. This may be related to the individual's personality and ability to accept responsibility or the new position may be beyond his intellectual capabilities. The nature of the job may create problems, e.g. a soldier in a war zone is under more stress than one in a training barracks. Lastly in times when unemployment is rife, job security is important and threats of redundancy may lead to anxiety at work. The results of work stress may be an anxiety state or depressive illness or may lead to the use of alcohol or minor tranquillizers, all of which may further affect the ability to cope with the job in hand.

Changes in the person doing the job

The first sign of intellectual decline may be an inability to cope with a job that has previously posed no problems though there have been no changes in the job itself. Impending dementia may also lead to a change in personality and behaviour. An acute psychosis may present initially as a crisis at work. Agoraphobia may cause problems travelling to work and obsessive compulsive neurosis with ritualistic behaviour may also affect work efficiency. Post-traumatic neuroses may affect work in general due to loss of self-esteem and self-confidence, or may lead to a phobic response to a specific job, as with a heavy goods vehicle driver who is involved in a road accident. Heavy drinking is associated with absenteeism, especially on a Monday, poor timekeeping, inefficiency and friction with other people at work. Poor timekeeping may also be due to domestic strife or illness, and psychotropic drugs may also affect efficiency at work. Finally isolated episodes of stealing from employers may equally reflect an acute psychiatric illness.

People at work

Any difficulties relating to people in general may manifest themselves primarily at work, which may be the only or commonest place where social intercourse occurs. There may be social anxiety, which might lead to inability to eat in the staff canteen or even to work refusal. On the other hand it may be part of a paranoid illness with ideas of persecution focused on all and sundry or on one person in particular. People who have difficulties relating to those in authority may have frequent and repeated problems with their foreman and managers at work.

Employment behaviour

Certain people may be chronically unable to hold down employment due to lack of intelligence, lack of volition as in chronic schizophrenia, regular intoxication with drugs or alcohol; or as a feature of a psychopathic personality disorder.

Social difficulties

People may present with an inability to cope with ordinary social situations, which may reflect a social phobia, or personality difficulties such as lack of self-esteem. Specific problems including physical deformity may contribute to social anxiety and are further discussed in Chapter 2. Paranoid ideation may also compromise normal social behaviour.

CASE HISTORY
EILEEN SIMPSON

Eileen Simpson, a 55-year-old divorced woman, was referred for an urgent psychiatric opinion by her general practitioner. She had been taken to see him by her daughter, who reported that over the last few days, Eileen, who was usually a cheerful, friendly and efficient lady, had seemed to have given up. She had stopped going to work (as a part-time shop assistant) three days before, was not doing her housework and was sitting at home, crying and shaking. Eileen said that she felt awful, but could not describe why; she had lost interest in everything, even in her daughter's three-month-old son to whom she had previously been devoted; she was feeling frightened and unhappy and could not concentrate on the simplest task. She could not give an account of her sleeping or eating over the last few days, but there was no apparent weight loss and she was well hydrated.

Eileen had no past psychiatric or medical history or family history of psychiatric illness. Her early life was happy and unremarkable. She had married, at the age of 20, a man who, after the first few years of marriage, was repeatedly adulterous, and whom she had divorced fifteen years before. She had two daughters from the marriage. The younger one, aged 25, had married and left home eighteen months ago and recently had her first child; she lived nearby and was on close terms with her mother. Her older daughter had died, at the age of 31, three years and two days before Eileen's visit to the GP. She had died from carcinoma of the breast and had been nursed by her mother in the last weeks of her illness. She left a husband and three young children who lived with Eileen for about a year after their mother's death. They had then moved away but remained in close contact with Eileen. About six weeks prior to the referral, Eileen's son-in-law had remarried; a woman whom she described as 'nice, really'.

Her GP said that she was an infrequent attender at the surgery; she had been prescribed benzodiazepines for a short time during and after her daughter's final illness, and exactly a year before, had sleeping tablets for about three weeks.

Eileen said that she remained very unhappy about the loss of her daughter, frequently thought of her and had never stopped missing her. She gave an account of how she and her son-in-law had grieved together for months after the death, and her daughter stated that her sister was frequently in their thoughts, was remembered with affection and pleasure and that her photograph remained on her mother's mantelpiece. The daughter said that she noticed her mother's deterioration after the previous weekend; she and her husband had planned to take her mother to the grave since it was the weekend nearest to the anniversary of her sister's death, but had postponed it because her husband's car had broken down.

Examination of Eileen's mental state revealed a thin, anxious woman who, although clean, had taken no pains with her appearance. She was perplexed and preoccupied, and concentrated poorly. She was hesitant and not spontaneous in her speech but was not retarded in movement. She gave a poor account of herself, saying she did not know how she felt and saying that she could not remember what had been happening. She agreed that her thoughts were of her daughter's death, and knew that the anniversary had just passed. She admitted to no suicidal ideas, and no abnormal beliefs and experiences were elicited. She was orientated for place and person, and for the time of day, but she was a day out in her assessment of the date and day of the week.

Questions

What is the differential diagnosis at the time of the first consultation and what is the immediate management?

What is the amended differential diagnosis by the time of the second consultation ten days later?

The evidence is that this disorder is of sudden onset, in a woman of previous good psychological health. There is a striking association of her symptoms with the anniversary of her daughter's death, and there is evidence of some disturbance the year before. Two other factors might explain why Mrs Simpson has broken down on this anniversary rather than previously: her son-in-law's remarriage with its inevitable effect on their previously close relationship; and her inability to visit the grave as arranged. A bereavement reaction is the likely diagnosis.

Mrs Simpson is depressed in mood but has no other evidence of a severe depressive illness. Her mental state is, however, curious in that she has severe difficulty in concentrating and is perplexed and preoccupied. The rapid onset, the apparent trigger of not being able to do what she wanted at the weekend, together with the fact that her daughter and her son-in-law are both preoccupied with their own families whilst she is left alone might indicate a hysterical or attention-seeking reaction, but hysteria is an exceedingly dangerous diagnosis to make for a disorder arising for the first time in middle or later life. The immediate management was agreed upon by the psychiatrist and the GP and Mrs Simpson's daughter. On the presumption that this was an abnormal grief reaction, it was arranged that Mrs Simpson would stay with her daughter and son-in-law, they would visit the grave the following weekend and the situation would be reassessed the following week.

The next appointment revealed new information. Mrs Simpson had no further complaints but was agitated and restless and did not apparently recognize the psychiatrist. Her daughter said that over the last few days her condition had varied; she had appeared more cheerful and communicative on occasion but at other times was vague and distant. She had cried on visiting the grave but had said little.

She had tried to return home after the weekend but had not been able to cope alone. She had not cooked and the flat had not been cleaned. In the few days she had been at home she had not washed or cared for herself at all, and she returned to live with her daughter. Even here, she had not eaten without prompting, and did not want to do anything that she normally enjoyed. She had, furthermore, asked where her bedroom was each night, had been incontinent of urine twice — The day before and that morning — and had not made any attempt to reach the lavatory. It was this that had prompted the earlier appointment with the doctor. She had started to write some Christmas cards (it was mid-December) but had become muddled and had written incoherent rubbish in several. Mrs Simpson remained orientated in place and person but now said she had no idea of the time.

Mrs Jones's state has deteriorated and the evidence now indicates that an organic state must be excluded. Incontinence of urine, especially when there seems little of the awareness of the need to urinate, should always alert one to the presence of an acute or chronic brain syndrome. Supportive evidence is that she was lost in her daughter's house and that she could not perform the relatively simple task of writing cards. An organic state also fits the pronounced failure of concentation and attention, but this diagnosis does not explain the association of psychological factors and the time of onset, and it is possible either that there are two diagnoses — organic brain disease plus an abnormal grief reaction — or that the timing is coincidental. A further possibility is that Mrs Simpson was already depressed either as a part of her organic brain pathology or as a reaction to this and thus was less able to cope with the psychological trauma of the anniversary of her daughter's death. A severe behavioural disorder, caused by Mrs Simpson's awareness of loneliness and of potential relative neglect by her family remains a possibility but cannot be primary diagnosis in the presence of pointers to an organic illness.

A further physical examination is mandatory, and an EEG is indicated. A CAT scan may be required, depending on the EEG result. In fact, bilateral early papilloedema was now evident, although Mrs Simpson continued to have no other neurological signs. Her EEG was abnormal; with pronounced high voltage delta and theta activity in the left frontotemporal region, indicating a strong likelihood of a left-sided space-occupying lesion. Surgery revealed a mass in her left frontal lobe, extending over the midline. Histology demonstrated a grade 4 glioblastoma multiforme; Mrs Simpson received radiotherapy but died ten months later.

9

Domestic violence

Physical violence within families is a phenomenon which is the proper concern of anthropologists and sociologists and, sometimes, psychiatrists. The precursors to violence in the home are complex and varied, and although the main factors are intrapersonal, for example, the inability to control or displace aggression, extrapersonal factors such as overcrowding, poverty and cultural 'norms' play a part. There is also variation in the levels that individual families set as 'acceptable' violence, some finding raised voices and broken teacups as intolerable whilst others tolerate actual physical harm. There is no doubt, too, that women in some cultures accept that it is normal to receive regular physical abuse from their husbands.

It is difficult, therefore, to specify what level of violence at home needs to be reached before it is viewed as a problem and hence made known to the outside world. For a working definition, life-threatening violence and abuse of those who cannot defend themselves should automatically be viewed as a problem requiring intervention; lesser degrees of violence expressed between equals may or may not be open to outside help. The inadequacy of this definition can be seen by the different attitudes to female circumcision in different cultures. In 'developed' societies this practice is universally condemned as an extreme example of violence against women; in some parts of the Third World it is commonly accepted as a normal cultural practice.

Attempts at classification of domestic violence into problem versus no problem are further defeated by variations in type and meaning of violence between intimates. Aggression and sexuality are particularly linked in violent outbursts between man and wife, and the level of pain tolerated during sexual behaviour varies between and within couples. Overtly violent sexual activities include rape of spouse and coerced incest. In other cases sexual aspects of violent behaviour are expressed more covertly. A further arbitrary distinction will be made between aggression and violence. We will consider acts of violence involving physical harm as distinct from those of aggression which are angry hostile acts which cause emotional, rather than physical harm.

VIOLENCE DIRECTED TOWARDS PARTICULAR FAMILY MEMBERS

1 Children.

Non-accidental injury

Child abuse is a severe problem, in its frequency, its extent, and the anxieties it causes as evidence of society's failure to protect its weakest members. It is said to be on the increase, with a frequency of 4,600 cases a year in the United Kingdom, but this assumption cannot be tested since detection depends entirely on the level of suspicion in those who come into contact with ill or injured children. All professionals involved in child care have become alert to this problem to an extent which would have been inconceivable 20 years ago.

All infants who have evidence of injury which cannot adequately be explained should be fully examined and radiologically screened if necessary. Bruises, abrasions, burns, scalds, cuts and fractures are common in non-accidental injury. Diagnosis is more difficult when parents deny abusing the child, but since such children are frequently victims of multiple attacks, evidence of old long bone fractures, resolving bruises etc., may be very important. Less obviously, minor injuries, together with failure to thrive and frequent admission to hospital for systemic illness, may point to child neglect as well as specific injury. For example, a child who died at 6 months of age from pneumonia had a history of four admissions to hospital with convulsions in the previous two months. The mother later confessed to habitually suffocating the baby with a polythene bag.

Child variables (Table 9.1) Children can be abused at all ages but are most frequently less than two years old at onset. They are often born prematurely and a high proportion of them have considerable neonatal morbidity which contributes to inadequate parental bonding. They are poorly stimulated and as a result are less wakeful at night, and lively during the day, than normal children, and may show developmental delay. Many people describe a state of 'frozen watchfulness' in affected children; the child is quiet, wary and alert to his surroundings, flinches or whimpers when approached and backs away from rather than moves towards others.

Abused children may be of either sex, though early studies showed a slight preponderance of boys. All siblings are at risk in abusing families, and there is a higher than expected child mortality, due in part to undiagnosed injury but also to other illnesses. This may be an index of the poorer health and social status of these children and their parents' general failure to recognize and respond to their needs. In some cases the abused child is mentally handicapped with severe behavioural problems. This may pose an intolerable level of stress on otherwise caring parents. Child abuse has a mortality of about 15% in most series, and a similar number of children are permanently disabled, usually neurologically, by their injuries.

Parental variables Although parents who deliberately harm their children are found in all types, ages, social classes and intelligence levels, several factors which are closely associated have been identified. These are youth, young maternal age in particular, low social class, low intelligence and abnormal personality. Most child injury inflicted by parents occurs as a result of loss of control of an explosive temper, and these parents show poor control of their temper in other situations. Mothers have inadequate understanding of the problems and satisfactions of child-rearing, and parents are likely to have been abused themselves as children. Many mothers are taking tranquillizers or antidepressants, many fathers have problems with alcohol abuse, and are unemployed. The combination of these parental problems with the health problems of the child (noted above) is the biggest predictor of risk. A minority of injured children are injured in bizarre ritualistic ways and this usually denotes serious mental illness in the parents. The majority of abusing parents, however, do not suffer from frank mental illness.

Infanticide

Infanticide is a legal term covering the killing of the child under twelve months of age by its mother, and was defined in the United Kingdom by an Act of Parliament in 1938. The Act recognizes that there are occasions when the mental health of the mother is such as to reduce her responsibility for the killing. Clearly many infanticides (in one series, about a third) occur as non-accidental injury as discussed above, but other causes are important.

Mothers who develop puerperal psychosis may kill their children for delusional reasons. The content of the abnormal beliefs usually demonstrates that an affected mother has not yet recognized the child as a separate entity but sees it as still a part of herself. Thus, fears of harm or damage to the child or fears that the mother or the child is possessed by the devil, or that they both

Table 9.1 Child and parental factors associated with non-accidental injury

child factors	Premature birth
	Neonatal illness
	Relatively unresponsive as infants
	Usually under 2 years when first abused
	Any sibling, either sex
	Mentally handicapped
Parental factors	Young maternal age
	Low intelligence
	Explosive or antisocial personality
	Socially and economically deprived
	Alcohol and drug abuse
	Experience of child abuse when themselves children

are causing terrible things to happen in the world, may precede the killing of the child and suicide of the mother. In epidemiological terms this is a minor problem compared with non-accidental injury, but it is of paramount clinical importance in the management of a mother who becomes psychotic in the puerperium. The child is usually subject to a slight act of violence and it is usually carried out as painlessly as possible, for example by suffocation.

Rarely, children born to isolated unsupported mothers are killed within hours or days of birth. Such mothers are often of sub-normal intelligence, have their babies alone and in secret, and are unable to cope with the consequences of an unplanned unwanted pregnancy.

Incest

Sexual relationships between family members other than spouses are subject to almost universal taboo. Because of condemnation by society, most incestuous activity does not come to attention, if at all, until years later. However, it is not uncommon in clinical practice for adult women to give a history of incest as a child, although it is difficult to be sure of the extent to which such experiencse are causally connected to curent problems. Sexual intercourse may occur between mother and son and brothers and sisters, although father-daughter incest is probably commonest. Daughters become subject to sexual abuse at any age but intercourse usually occurs after the age of ten and may continue throughout adolescence. As the daughter becomes older and refuses to continue to comply, the father may turn to the abuse of younger siblings. Incest is a problem for the whole family and the wife and mother often colludes with the activity although she may deny awareness that it occurs. Incest may be admitted to by the family in a crisis; when for example the father presents with symptoms of depression, anxiety or alcohol abuse; and should be suspected in adolescent girls who run away from home and say they are frightened to return, but will not elaborate further.

Incest is a criminal offence and social service departments have statutory responsibilities to protect children from sexual as well as from any

other abuse. Imprisonment is, however, rarely a therapeutic move in dealing with the problem.

2 Spouse

Violence between spouses usually involves the wife as victim, and husband as perpetrator, although it does occur vice versa. Women tend to be less strong and express their aggression in less physical ways. The term 'battered wife' has been defined as repeated deliberate injuries inflicted by the husband and does not encompass individual acts of rage and aggression. The frequency of such cases is unknown, but since the establishment of refuges for victims, more women admit to being subject to violence from their husbands. Families with this pattern of violence show similarities to child-abusing families and indeed the two phenomena may coexist, both with the husband perpetrating violence on wife and children and by wives taking out their feelings by hitting the children after they themselves have been attacked. Violent husbands have frequently been victims of violence in their childhood; personality disorder and alcohol abuse are common in both partners, but serious mental illness uncommon. All social classes are represented. Jealousy is a significant factor (see below). Injuries are usually around the head, and fists or weapons may be used.

The victim of marital violence tends to have low self-esteem which antedates the violence and indicates that she has low expectations of the respect due to her. She is frequently overwhelmed by her domestic responsibilities, sees no way of living independently from her husband and is trapped in a dangerous relationship. A minority of victims are provocative, both sexually and otherwise, and such a woman may taunt her husband until his violence is unleashed; such women repeatedly enter relationships where they become the victims of violence. Very occasionally victims of violence are frankly mentally ill, e.g. manic, and the severe behavioural disturbance provokes explosive violence in the spouse.

Rape of spouse.

The criminal offence of rape occurs if a man has sexual intercourse with a woman who at the time does not consent to it, and he knows that she does not. On this definition it is obvious that rape can occur within marriage, and there is clinical and anecdotal evidence that is occurs fairly commonly in marriages where there is little mutual respect and frequent violence. However the current legal position in England and Wales is that a man can only be convicted of the rape of his wife if they are legally separated.

3 The Elderly

Many frail elderly people are cared for by their relatives who show devotion to them. Elderly demented people can create enormous strain for their spouses and children by their erratic behaviour and increasing dependence, and by the restriction on the family's activities which may continue for years. Tolerance by families depends to a large measure on the balance between love and duty, and on the quality of relationships between the generations. Frustration, resentment and exhaustion may explode into violence against the elderly person, often as a result of a 'last straw' such as another episode of incontinence or wandering in the night. Unspoken fears of such behaviour may underlie the sudden refusal of a relative to have an elderly parent home from hospital, despite a history of caring; professionals involved in the care of the elderly should be alert to signs that families are stretched to breaking point, since elderly people are vulnerable to injury, out of proportion to the violence displayed. In recent years too, there have been examples of deliberate and malicious emotional and physical harm to defenceless elderly relatives for gain although such planned exploitation is rare.

PSYCHIATRIC DISORDERS ASSOCIATED WITH DOMESTIC VIOLENCE

Personality Disorders

The extent to which aggression and violence form part of the emotional response of an individual depends on his/her personality structure. This is determined by genetic and environmental factors, both intrapersonal and cultural. Some disorders of personality development are characterized by aggressive antisocial behaviour and are classified as psychopathic or sociopathic disorders. Their characteristic features include intense egocentricity, inability to delay the satisfaction of immediate wants and needs, inability to learn from experience, and perhaps most importantly in this context, a deficient or absent sense of conscience. Such persons may resort to violence as a means of obtaining their own way, often on minor issues, and will show very low tolerance of frustration. They often come from families where violence is a major method of communication, and aggression and violence persistently characterize their own dealings with others. Alternatively there are explosive personalities whose violence is intermittently displayed. Since those with whom one lives closely may well be those most likely to cause one frustration and assert their own needs in competition with one's own, persons with psychopathic personality disorders frequently involve their familes in their violence. However, this is usually non-specific and many violent episodes occasioned by these individuals occur at work, in the pub, on the football terraces and randomly on the street. Many violence, often wth fatal consequences, may occur as an isolated incident in overcontrolled personalities. In these people, the normal self-assertive response to domestic discord is buried beneath obsessional defences, and after years of mute acceptance, a relatively minor incident may provoke uncontrollable rage.

Alcohol And Drug Abuse

Alcoholism is strongly associated with violence for many reasons. It is a cerebral depressant but acts initially to disinhibit, so that intoxication is likely to release aggression from internal controls. People who frequently become drunk, through either alcohol dependence or heavy social drinking, are at risk, and domestic violence is most likely to occur in this context. Alcoholics also deteriorate in their standards of personal behaviour, may develop paranoid psychoses — especially delusions of infidelity (see below) — and suffer brain damage which increases disinhibition. Similarly drug abuse may lead to violence, as a result either of acute intoxication or of chronic paranoid psychosis.

Any individual dependent on alcohol, drugs or activities such as gambling may resort to violence as a means of obtaining money and resources to finance his needs. If an individual's priorities are rearranged so that pursuit of, say, money for gambling is the most important motivation in his life, then other issues, such as respect and affection for family members, may be so lacking in priority that they are discounted. There is obviously a strong connection between this type of behaviour and the psychopathic personality disorders described above.

Morbid Jealousy (see Table 9.2)

Jealousy is a common emotion between close individuals; the point at which it becomes pathological or morbid depends both on its form and on its intensity. Some insecure individuals are chronically worried that their partners will leave them, but they may be able to keep this fear to themselves. In others, however, the jealousy dominates their every act; they will constantly question their partner, follow him or her around and can never be reassured; this jealousy is morbid. It is important to remember that this condition is not a diagnosis in itself (although often termed the Othello syndrome), but a symptom of many different conditions.

Neurotic jealousy occurs in people with anxious, paranoid personalities who have low self-esteem, and project this sense on to others. They expect to be rejected and abandoned and behave in clinging possessive ways to their intimates, most especially their sexual partners. They may behave violently in this context but are able to see the irrationality of their fears. This type of behaviour, however, is not compatible with stable relationships and frequently provokes the rejection which is feared.

Delusional jealousy is a psychotic condition where the patient believes, incorrigibly and against rational evidence, in the infidelity of his partner. It is the irrational basis from which the belief is drawn which points to the diagnosis — a belief system is constructed on evidence which would not normally be taken as relevant. For example a patient may say, 'I knew my wife was unfaithful when she started to wear nylon stockings and not tights.' Patients with delusional jealousy behave in increasingly suspicious ways; examining their bedroom linen and spouses underwear for stains; checking up on their every movement, laying traps for them and interpreting everyday behaviour as evidence of unfaithfulness.

The person may have other paranoid ideas: for example, that the partner has tried to poison him or given him something to reduce his sexual potency. Sometimes the ideas are bizarre in the extreme: for example, accusations that the imaginary lover has got into the bedroom through the keyhole and the partner has had intercourse with him while the patient has been asleep even though they have both been sharing the same bed.

Delusional jealousy is a paranoid psychotic state and may form part of a schizophrenic illness, or a more circumscribed paraphrenic condition, or it may be the only abnormality as in a monosymptomatic delusional psychosis.

Morbid jealousy is frequently associated with alcoholism. Insecure jealous men are prone to drink excessively, and alcoholism will exacerbate a pre-existing personality trait. Alcoholics who develop a paranoid psychosis, hallucinosis or dementia, are liable to become delusional in their jealousy. Sexual jealousy is exacerbated by impotence, which is frequent in alcoholic men. Delusional jealousy may be a symptom of a depressive illness, although depression is frequently secondary to the jealousy and it may be difficult to decide which condition came first. Organic brain disease may also give rise to morbid jealousy.

Morbid jealousy is a highly important cause of extreme domestic violence, especially when it is persistent and intractable. The condition is most common between men and their wives though sometimes other relatives may be significantly at

Table 9.2 Psychiatric diagnosis associated with jealousy

Neurotic jealousy	Anxiety states
	Paranoid personality disorder
	Sensitive, insecure personality
Delusional jealousy	Schizophrenia
	Paranoid states
	Monosymptomatic delusional psychosis
	Alcohol dependence
	Depressive illness
	Dementia

risk from attack. The dangerousness of the condition is that violence may be premeditated, extreme, and murderous. The safety of the spouse must always be considered when cases of morbid jealousy present.

Grief Reactions

The failure of a relationship is frequently accompanied by rows, recriminations and a search for revenge, especially when the relationship breaks up because one partner leaves to live with someone else. The rejected person may act out his or her jealousy and vengefulness on either the old partner, the new lover or both, and this may be a sudden impulsive act or a carefully laid plan. Extreme fatal violence may ensue and may be followed by suicide. Such acts, although newsworthy, are rare, and are most likely to be perpetrated by extremely dependent individuals who have idolized their partner and who have failed to perceive, or adjust to, the evidence that their relationshiup has been failing

Sadomasochism

Physical abuse and injury may be inflicted on sexual partners by individuals whose sexual satisfaction is heightened by giving and receiving pain. Sexual perversions are considered in chapter 6 but a brief mention of sadomasochism is relevant here. Sexual satisfaction for sadomasochists, is attained through a wide range of abnormal behaviours encompassing all degrees of emotional and physical abuse, from verbal taunts and humiliations through to serious physical harm. Most sadomasochists are gratified by both the active and passive aspects of this practice, and many sadomasochistic men are impotent without this stimulus. When both partners are consenting, problems may only arises when errors occur causing more severe injuries than anticipated; but it must be borne in mind that many cases of apparent consent involve coercion or worse by the dominant partner. Sadomasochistic practices are often ritualized and should be suspected in cases of injury to the erogenous zones where explanations as to the cause are bizarre or incomplete.

Depression

Severely depressed patients may harm their loved ones and themselves under delusional beliefs that dreadful harm is to come to the family, that the world is about to end, or that the depressed patient has irrevocably damaged the lives of all the family so that death is the only solution. There is no conscious pleasure in the attack which is usually designed to kill as quickly and painlessly as possible, and to be followed by the suicide of the perpetrator. This behaviour is uncommon but its risk should be noted if a depressed patient talks of beliefs and anxieties of the type described above. Multiple domestic murders followed by suicide are the usual outcome, although some or all of the victims may escape death, depending on the efficiency of the patient and the lethality of the method chosen.

Mania

Manic patients are dangerous to those around them because their judgment is impaired: as, for example, the patient who drove his car at 60 mph on the pavement because it was quicker than driving on the road. In addition, they may become aggressive when their wishes are thwarted and their limited tolerance is exceeded. The disinhibiting effect of mania may permit the expression of violent hatred in families where there is pre-existing discord.

Schizophrenia

Contrary to popular belief the vast majority of schizophrenic patients are not violent. They may, however, act violently in self-defence against presumed aggressors; subjects either of their delusional beliefs or of their hallucinatory experiences. Such attacks will usually be unprovoked, and not understandable in the absence of knowledge of the patient's psychotic world. There is no particular likelihood that such attacks will involve family members, except where these members are involved in the patient's delusional system. Violent episodes in schizophrenic patients are difficult to predict, but care should be taken when accounts of increasing irritability, hostility and preoccupation are given by relatives. This may particularly be true where mothers report fear of their schizophrenic sons. Matricide is an uncommon crime, but overwhelmingly committed by sons, most of whom have a diagnosis of schizophrenia.

Organic Disorder

Acute confusional states

Patients who are delirious may mistake family members for jailors or other persecutors, and may hit out in self-defence. They are usually too disorientated and ill to design and carry through a motivated act of aggression but may harm those around them by, for example, throwing heavy objects at them.

Dementia

Demented patients, the vast majority of whom are cared for at home, may cause unintentional harm to those who care for them, especially if the principal carer is an elderly frail spouse. Patients with dementia who are deluded that for example, their father is alive but they are prevented from seeing him, may threaten and hit others in their anger, but harmful behaviour more often results from kicking, scratching and biting others, rather in the way that a frustrated child does when in a temper tantrum.

Epilepsy

There is an association between epilepsy and psychiatric disturbance. A schizophrenia-like psychosis may occur with temporal lobe (complex-partial) epilepsy, usually succeeding the onset of epilepsy by many years. Repeated anoxia from ictal episodes may cause cognitive deterioration and personality changes may occur. In addition, epileptic patients may have grave difficulties in emotional and social adjustments, and are discriminated against to some extent in many societies. Thus there are many reasons why epileptic patients may have difficulties in their personal lives and thus become at risk of involvement in a relationship characterized by tension, unhappiness, hostility and perhaps violence. It is not true, however, to say that epilepsy *per se* predisposes to

violence, and many studies support the fact that there is not a strong association between violent behaviour and epilepsy. This is particularly so in the case of automatism. Automatism occurs in ictal or post-ictal phases and usually lasts a few minutes only; the patient carries out apparently purposeful acts without awareness. Automatisms are not common and the behaviours exhibited during them are almost always mundane and ordinary; violent behaviour in automatism is extremely rare.

The Neuroses

In neurotic disorders aggression directed to other members of the family is most often passive and verbal. However, physical violence can occur, especially if a spouse ceases to collude with, or accept, the patient's neurotic behaviour. For example, if a husband of an agoraphobic housewife refuses to do the shopping for the family, or the wife of an obsessional man stops reassuring him that he did count to 100, and not to 99, before getting up in the morning, violent threats and actions may result when verbal coercion fails.

CASE HISTORY

BARRY SMITH

Mr Barry Smith, a 46-year-old builder, attended psychiatric outpatients with his wife Marjorie. He came reluctantly, and said he had come at the insistence of his GP whom he trusted, and preferred to be interviewed alone. He did not think there was anything wrong with him apart from the stress and worry caused by his marital difficulties. His wife had, he said, been having an affair with a man at work (she was a typist in a large office) for about a year and although she denied this, she had on one occasion, about a month ago, admitted that she was unfaithful. He said that he was still in love with her but these days they were always arguing about her 'affair' and he often became physically violent — usually breaking things in the home, but on one occasion he had hit her.

Mr Smith was the middle one of five siblings with whom he retained little contact. His parents had a poor relationship; they had separated several times for short periods throughout their marriage and Mr Smith remembered his home as unhappy, tense and characterized by rows. He had a stable employment record, but often had arguments at work over being 'put on' by the others, and had been prosecuted for assault at the age of twenty-five after a fight at work.

He had married his wife twenty years ago when she was pregnant with their first daughter. The marriage had been 'up and down', and they had separated for six months after the birth of their second daughter fifteen years ago. During this time they both had affairs with other partners but he had eventually effected a reconciliation. He admitted he had always been possessive of his wife, he was extremely proud of her attractiveness but did not like going out to dances and clubs, whilst she did.

Mr Smith first began to doubt his wife's fidelity about a year before when she extended her part-time hours at work. He now believed this was so that she could spend more time with her lover. He had become sure of her infidelity about nine months previously, when he phoned her at work to be told that she was not there but had taken an early lunch. On her return from work she had told him that she had gone shopping but had not seen anything she liked and come back empty-handed. He became angry and accused her of having an affair; she laughed at him. From that time on he had become preoccupied with obtaining proof; and felt he had confirmed her infidelity one day when she wore a dress to work which was shorter than usual. Three months ago he had arrived home from work early to find that the bed linen was included in a load of washing and he knew she had been entertaining her lover that afternoon. His daughters supported their mother and would not admit the 'truth' to him, even though he pleaded with them.

Mr Smith said that this had made him very depressed. It had affected his work; his sleep was restless and interrupted. He had very recently lost his interest in sex, but he said that his wife had refused him intercourse for about a year. He admitted that he 'liked a drink' in the past and had been in the habit of drinking five or six pints of beer most nights.

He was angry, suspicious and defensive throughout the interview. He was in no doubt that his wife was unfaithful and said that any other interpretation of his wife's behaviour meant that she had fooled everyone else too. He was aggrieved and self-pitying. There were no other mental state abnormalities.

The interview with his wife alone indicated a rather different picture. She denied ever being unfaithful and said her daughters knew the truth; she had had no affair during the separation from her husband but she had left him to live with her parents because of his drunken, inconsiderate behaviour. She had initially been rather pleased by his pride and possessiveness until she realized that he could not tolerate her having a life of her own. She felt the problem had really begun eight years before when she first started work, and had become worse when she began to have a night out with the girls once a week. He had been, throughout their marriage, frequently drunk. Their sexual life had always been unsatisfactory to her and she had been relieved when three years before his demands had begun to decline in frequency; she supposed that they had had intercourse only four or five times in the previous year. She admitted that she had, in desperation, said that she was having an affair because she was exhausted by constant questioning; she regretted that immediately. She said that she had realized her husband was ill when, two weeks before, he had accused her of putting sleeping tablets in his tea so that she could entertain her lover whilst he slept.

Questions

What are the pathological aspects of Mr Smith's jealousy?
What aetiological factors are identifiable?
What is your immediate management?

Mr Smith's jealousy is morbid; his has always been a jealous and possessive nature, but his current state is beyond the bounds of normality, both quantitatively and qualitatively. He is preoccupied with suspicions of his wife to the exclusion of work and social activity, and most of his home conversation is dominated by it. More importantly, the nature of his belief is delusional. To have come back empty-handed from a shopping trip is not, in itself, a rational basis for a belief of infidelity, and neither is the wearing of particular clothes, nor Mrs Smith's washing of bed linen. Note that it is not whether the belief is true or not which makes it delusional; it is the evidence on which the belief is based which is important. Mrs Smith may indeed be having an affair, particularly since she may feel that she is going to be accused of it anyway she may as well; but that does not call the diagnosis into question since Mr Smith bases his belief system on evidence which would not rationally be associated with the presence or absence of fidelity.

The aetiology can only be provisional at this stage; further assessment will be required for a firm diagnosis. There is no evidence that this is paranoid schizophrenia; there are no abnormal perceptions, thought disorders or abnormal beliefs in other areas. Although he is depressed there is little evidence at this stage of a primary major depressive episode, nor is there any evidence of an organic state. A fuller assessment of Mr Smith's alcohol history will be required before the differentiation between alcoholic jealousy (ICD–9 281.5) and simple paranoid state (ICD–9 297.0) can be made.

There are several potentially important aetiological factors. Mr Smith's early experience of inconsistent, unhappy family life may be an important cause of his insecurity. He has always been rather suspicious and prickly, and his relationship with his wife is one of insecure attachment. He is chronically jealous and the development of his illness may have been influenced by his wife's first move to independence and by his declining sexual potency — itself possibly due to alcohol dependence.

Immediate management would ideally be to admit Mr Smith to psychiatric hospital for full investigation and assessment, but it is unlikely that he has sufficient insight to agree to that. He may interpret the suggestion as aimed at allowing his wife more freedom. The situation is potentially dangerous, however, to Mrs Smith and their daughters, and possibly even to her male colleagues at work. Mr. Smith is a violent and aggressive man, who drinks to excess and whose condition is becoming worse; further assessment must be made to ascertain whether his dangerousness warrants detention under the Mental Health Act 1983.

10

Breaking the law

Psychiatry comes into contact with the law in four broad areas: firstly the psychiatric assessment of people who have committed crimes; secondly in family and custody issues; thirdly in civil law — compensation cases, negligence and court of protection; and lastly in the working of the Mental Health Act.

CRIMINAL LAW

Many research projects have highlighted the high level of mental disorder in prisons, and most general adult psychiatrists have as part of their clinical role the task of preparing on opinion on the psychiatric state of people who have committed crimes. Important issues on which an opinion is usually sought are fitness to plead, criminal responsibility, level of dangerousness and disposal. Though the majority of offenders are not psychiatrically ill there is a sizeable minority to whom a psychiatric diagnostic label can be attached. Common diagnoses include schizophrenia, drug and alcohol abuse and psychopathic personality disorder, though the relative frequency of these and associated disorders differs according to the crime committed.

THE LEGAL PROCESS

As noted above three of the areas on which a psychiatrist is asked to give an opinion are fitness to plead, criminal responsibility and dangerousness.

Fitness to plead

In order to be classed as fit to plead the defendant has to satisfy the following criteria:
1 He must understand the nature of the charge.
2 He must understand the difference between pleading guilty and not guilty.
3 He must be able to instruct counsel.
4 He must be able to challenge jurors.
5 He must be able to follow the evidence present in court.

Criminal responsibility.

To be guilty of an offence a person must have both carried out the offence — *actus rea*; and have had the intention of so doing — *mens rea*. The *McNaughton rules* were the criteria initially used for deciding whether a murderer was responsible for his actions. These stated that he was not responsible if: either he did not know the nature and quality of his actions or: he did know these but did not know that what he was doing was wrong. The plea was not guilty because of insanity. For various reasons these criteria were not felt to be adequate and the concept of *diminished responsibility* was introduced for those situations where the accused was suffering from an abnormality of mind such as to have substantially impaired his mental responsibility for his acts and omissions. Though this term is only used for charges of murder the concept on which it is based can be applied to any other offence. Finally if a crime is committed when the person is unaware of what he is doing and has no control over his actions then he is not guilty due to *automatism*.

Automatism may be due to hypoglycaemia or sleepwalking, but where it is due to a disease of the mind then the person is found not guilty because of insanity. This is at present the legal position regarding epileptic automatism.

Dangerousness

One issue on which the psychiatrist is often called to comment is the risk of future dangerousness posed by the defendant. With increasing levels of violence in psychiatric hospitals this issue is also relevant to the non-forensic clinical setting. Predictors for future dangerousness of somebody who has carried out a violent act are set out in Table 10.1; however, the prediction of an indi-

Table 10.1 Predictors of dangerousness

Offence	bizarre violence (quality better predictor of violence than quantity)
	presence of continuing adverse factors, e.g. drugs and alcohol, bad companions
	lack of remorse
	continuing denial
	lack of provocation
	failure to consider solutions other than violence
Past history	previous violent offences
	early history of aggressive behaviour
	childhood deprivation
	abnormal personality traits — paranoid, sadomasochistic, deceptive, jealous
	Impulsive behaviour
	Inability to cope with stress
	Inability to delay gratification
	Poor self-control
Personal data	male sex
	youth
	never satisfactory sexual relationships
	poor social circumstances
	lack of support
Mental state	paranoid delusions accompanied by a wish to act on them
	morbid jealousy
	poor attitude to treatment
	threats to repeat violence
Circumstances after the offence	Continuing presence of precipitants or stresses
	continuing presence of adverse factors (see above)
	lack of social support

vidual's future dangerousness remains a very difficult and imprecise judgment.

CRIMES OF VIOLENCE

Homicide

A person charged with homicide is more likely to be male, often in the twenties or early thirties, with the victim frequently known and/or related to him. In one study of murderers, fifty per cent were normal; twenty-five per cent had psychopathic personality disorders; and twenty per cent were psychotic — the vast majority being schizophrenic. The remaining five per cent were of subnormal intelligence. Female murderers were more likely to be mentally ill than male murderers, and alcohol was an element in fifty per cent of all male murders. Motiviating circumstances included arguments, delusions, robbery and sexual crime.

Homicide followed by suicide

About ten per cent of murderers commit suicide following their crime. This group is distinguished demographically from the rest by the increased proportion of women, the higher social class of offenders, the smaller number of previous convictions and the increased incidence of psychiatric illness. Severe puerperal psychosis carries an increased risk of infanticide followed by suicide; a similar sequence of events may occur in either party after the break-up of a relationship or as a result of depression, and may involve one or more members of the family.

SEXUAL OFFENCES

Rape

This is defined as intercourse without consent. Though force is often used it is not a necessary constitituent of the crime. In one classic study of rapists it was found that they could be categorized in three groups. Fifty per cent were rapists with few if any other convictions, and included young men who misinterpreted the partner's signals as consent. In twenty per cent the act was overtly violent and there was a history of aggressive offences, not necessarily sexual in nature, and of heavy drinking. In the remaining thirty per cent the offence was paedophilic rape.

When compared with other sexual offenders, rapists tend to have less overt psychiatric disease and fewer previous sexual offences. The most common diagnostic subgroup is antisocial personality disorder although subnormal intelligence must also be considered. Homosexual rape occurs, although with less frequency except in exclusively male institutions such as prisons.

Paedophilia

Paedophiliacs engage or wish to to engage in sexual activity with prepubertal children. They are almost exclusively male and the relationship may be a heterosexual or homosexual one. Paedophiliacs include young men with overinhibited, frustrated personality traits as well as older and more deviant offenders. Psychiatric diagnoses include inadequate or psychopathic personalities, subnormal intelligence or organic and functional psychoses in which the person is unaware of what he is doing or is acting in response to delusions or hallucinations.

Indecent exposure (Exhibitionism)

This is the deliberate display of genital and/or other sexual areas in an inappropriate situation. There are two main diagnostic categories of exhibitionists. Firstly, there are inhibited young men, often of a shy and anxious personality, who have a compulsion to expose themselves. The act is often accompanied by extreme anxiety and tension which may be relieved by the behaviour. In some cases exposing is all that happens but subsequently the patient may masturbate to memories of the act. Psychiatric and clinical data for this group suggest that the patients have immature, passive and obsessional personalities with poor self-control. The risk of offending is increased with life stresses and depression. Such exhibitionists come from families with overprotective, dominant mothers, and fathers who are either passive and ineffectual or harsh and brutal. They tend to have stable marriages in which they behave childishly, are ambivalent and dependent on their wives, with fewer children than other men, perhaps because they see them as rivals for the wife's (mother's) attention. There are often other psychosexual problems such as dissatisfaction with sexual appearance and sexual dysfunction including impotence and premature ejaculation. Other offences are rare in this group.

The second group consists of peope with antisocial personalities who expose with an erect penis and derive great pleasure from frightening their victims. Exposure may also be associated with more overt sexual contact, when the risk of further serious sexual offences is increased.

Prostitution

According to the Street Offences Act 1959, of the activities involved in prostitution, only soliciting is illegal. It has been estimated that six per cent of women in prison are there because of offences of prostitution, but that a quarter to a third have been prostitutes at one time in their life. Prostitution is not infrequently associated with drug and alcohol abuse, and a past psychiatric history including attempted suicide and concurrent physical disorder. Sexual orientation is often homosexual or bisexual.

CHILD STEALING

Women who steal children may do so to gain comfort, e.g., following a stillbirth or miscarriage; in order to manipulate circumstances; or impulsively in the presence of psychiatric illness, e.g., subnormality, schizophrenia, or psychopathic personality disorder. There has been no major psychiatric study of child stealing in men, though they are more commonly charged with this offence.

DOMESTIC VIOLENCE (see Chapter 9)

ACTUAL AND GREVIOUS BODILY HARM

Psychiatrically, this is most likely to be associated with personality disorders especially of the psychopathic or antisocial type with paranoid or sadistic traits and associated with drug and alcohol abuse, or with paranoid psychoses including schizophrenia as a response to delusions and/or hallucinations. The issue of dangerousness commonly occurs with these patients (see table 10.1).

CRIMES AGAINST PROPERTY

Shoplifting

Shoplifting has of recent years become known as the crime of the middle-aged, depressed woman. Though this may be true in certain circumstances the vast majority of shoplifters steal for gain. Nevertheless, where psychiatric illness is present, it is often depression, in women generally of previously good character, with a low rate of reconviction; and the motivation may include self-punishment and a cry for help. Chronic schizophrenics, alcoholics and drug absuers may shoplift because of lack of money. Confused or demented patients, those of subnornmal intelligence and those with high levels of arousal, for example, in phobic anxiety states or during a hysterical dissociative state, and those under the influence of alcohol or drugs, including psychotropic drugs, may simply forget to pay. Shoplifting may also occur in acute schizophrenia and mania, where the behaviour is usually part of the psychosis. In juveniles such offences may be carried out to show off and obtain approval from the peer group, to buy friends or as 'comfort' stealing.

Arson

Some arsonists light fires for financial gain, others for political motives, for revenge, or as part of an act of homicide. In some there is evidence of psychiatric illness, mental retardation or alcohol abuse, while others light fires for the fire's sake alone, either for sexual gratification or in order to be seen as a hero by helping the fire brigade put the fire out. Where psychiatric illness is present this may be an organic or functional psychosis, and the act may be in some cases part of a suicide as in self-immolation, or it my be a cry for help. Arson may also be committed while the person is under the influence of drugs or alcohol.

Criminal Damage

Criminal damage is one of the commonest crimes committed by people referred for a psychiatric opinion. Not infrequently the crime is committed while the person is under the influence of alcohol or drugs; as part of a personality disorder where he is unable to tolerate frustation; or as a response to paranoid delusions and/or hallucinations.

PSYCHIATRIC ILLNESS AND CRIMINALITY

Psychoses

Schizophrenia

Schizophrenia is over-represented in crimes of violence although most schizophrenics are not violent, and when they come into conflict with the law this is usually because of crimes of lesser magnitude due to the general deterioration in their level of social functioning.

Affective disorders

Depression is rarely associated with violence towards others though it may occur in the presence of depressive delusions where the crime, often homicide, may be followed by attempted or completed suicide. This is further discussed in Chapter 9. Crimes against property are also sometimes associated with depression as in shop lifting in middle-aged women. Depression may lead to alcohol abuse which is itself frequently associated with crime.

Grief reactions

These can sometimes be of such severity as to lead to homicide or suicide. This is especially true where the grief reaction is the result of the break-up of a relationship, and it is important when assessing these patients to ask about ideas of homicide as well as suicides.

Mania

Manic patients may come into conflict with the law either because of violence due to irritability and aggressive behaviour, or following spending sprees without the finances to back them up.

Paranoid psychoses

People with paranoid psychoses, whatever their aetiology, are especially prone to violent behaviour.

Organic psychoses

Violence may occur as a result of paranoid ideation and heightened level of arousal in patients with acute confusional states. On the other hand demented patients may commit minor offences due to failing memory and disintegrating personality; occasionally this may lead to sexual offences.

Epilepsy

The incidence of epilepsy amongst prisoners is higher than that in the general population. Temporal lobe epilepsy and temporal lobe brain damage (even without epilepsy) may be associated with aggressive behaviour. Criminal acts may be carried out during the psychomotor seizure itself or during the post-ictal confusional state. According to a recent ruling, if a crime is committed during these periods then the plea is one of insane automatism.

Morbid Jealousy

This is a disorder in which one partner in a relationship becomes preoccupied with the other's fidelity. In some cases this leads to violence including murder which may be followed by suicide. This is further discussed in Chapter 9.

Personality Disorder (see Table 10.2)

The assessment of personality disorder has been dealt with briefly in Chapter 1. In ICD–9 the definition of personality disorder is: 'Deeply ingrained maladaptive patterns of behaviour, generally recognizable by the time of adolescence or earlier, and continuing throughout most of adult life although often becoming less obvious in middle or old age. The personality is abnormal whether in the balance of its components, their

Table 10.2 Classification of personality disorders

ICD–9	DSM–III
301.0 Paranoid	Paranoid
301.1 Affective	*
301.2 Schizoid	Schizoid Schizotypal 301.22
301.3 Explosive	**
301.4 Anankastic	Compulsive
301.5 Hysterical	Histronic
301.6 Asthenic	Dependent
301.7 Personality disorder with predominantly sociopathic or asocial manifestations	Antisocial
301.8 Other: includes passive-aggressive	Narcissistic 301.81 Avoidant 308.82 Borderline 301.83 Passive-Aggressive 301.84 Atypical, Mixed or other 301.89
301.9 Unspecified	

* Classified in DSM–III under affective disorders as Cyclothymic Disorder 301.13
** Classified in DSM–III under disorders of Impulse Control 312

quality and expression or in its total aspect. Because of this deviation or psychopathology the patient suffers or others have to suffer and there is adverse effect upon the individual or on society'. The DSM–III, which includes in the diagnosis an axis of personality disorder, defines this as: 'Deeply ingrained, inflexible maladaptive patterns of relating to, perceiving and thinking about the environment and oneself which are of sufficient severity to cause either significant impairment in adaptive functioning or subjective distress'.

Both the ICD–9 and DSM–III subdivide personalities into a classificatory system or different descriptive subgroups; these number more in DSM–III than in ICD–9. Psychologists view personality in a different schematic way, using personality inventories to measure personality on various dimensions rather than creating descriptive subgroups. Many patients with severe personality disorders are not classifiable according to any one specific group but show signs of traits that are pertinent to a number of different groups.

Patients with personality disorders may come up against the law in the following ways.

Paranoid personality

These people are usually sensitive and suspicious. They may be jealous and suffer from morbid jealousy, or they may aggressively defend their 'rights' which may lead to excessive litigation regardless of the merits of their case. Violence may occur, often associated with alcohol abuse.

Affective personality

These people suffer from a lifelong abnormality of mood not severe enough to warrant the diagnosis of an affective illness. This mood may be one of depression, or of elation, or may swing from one to the other (cyclothymic personality). They are most likely to come into conflict with the law as a result of drinking in response to mood.

Schizoid personality

This describes a withdrawal from socializing, with marked introspection, coolness and detachment. Occasionally this is associated with sexually deviant behaviour, sometimes criminal and sadistic in nature.

Explosive personality

This is characterized by uncontrollable outbursts of aggression, either physical or verbal, against a background which is not otherwise antisocial in nature.

Anankastic (compulsive) personality

This is characterized by rigidity, compulsiveness and obsessionality. People with this personality may be overcontrolled and slow to express anger, but the final loss of control can lead to disaster as in the case of the long-suffering wife who murders her husband following intolerable harrassment.

Hysterical or histrionic personality

Patients with this personality are demanding and attention-seeking with a theatrical quality to the way they present and behave. Despite outwardly appearing to be highly emotionally and sexually aroused, they are usually emotionally shallow with difficulties in making meaningful relationships. They may turn to drink or drugs or petty crime to attract attention.

Asthenic or dependent personality

This is characterized by an inability to cope with normal demands of everyday life, with marked dependency and inadequacy. This may lead to alcohol abuse, indulgence in petty crime or domestic violence.

Antisocial personality

People with this personality are commonly known as psychopaths or sociopaths and show antisocial behaviour with a lack of conscience, an inability to learn from mistakes, a history of failure in work and relationships; yet often have a superficial charm which may make them attractive to the onlooker who does not suffer from their antisocial behaviour. There is usually a history of inadequate parenting, juvenile deliquency with disturbed behaviour at school, lying, petty theft, alcohol and drug abuse. The antisocial behaviour itself may be of an irresponsible or seriously aggressive type, when the violence may be sadistic and callous with no remorse. They represent probably the most difficult group of patients for the forensic psychiatrist to deal with, because whereas society deems them to be in need of psychiatric treatment, they do not respond to this and many psychiatrists feel they should be treated as 'bad' rather than 'mad'.

Narcissistic personality

These people with severe disturbance of personality structure are grandiose and self-important as a defence against fears of not existing. Their behaviour may be attention-seeking, may involve drug or alcohol abuse, and may become antisocial.

Borderline personality

This is a term used to describe a group of people who show transient psychotic and neurotic symptoms without being classifiable under either heading. There may be shortlived episodes of depression, sometimes associated with anger and aggression. Impulsive behaviour may also lead them into conflict with the law as may alcohol and drug abuse.

Passive-aggressive personality

This term is used for people who underachieve by responding to requests for performance with a perverse and intentional failure to do so by means within the person's control. In certain circumstances, for example, under the influence of alcohol, they may be involved in minor crime.

Neuroses

People with phobic anxiety states may be so over-aroused as to fail to act appropriately in certain situations; for example, they may not pay for goods bought in shops. This may be due to the cerebral response to anxiety interfering with concentration or a panic attack leading to leaving the shop without paying. Psychotropic drugs may affect intellect, behaviour and memory. Crimes may be committed during hysterical dissociative states with subsequent amnesia for the episodes.

Subnormality

Patients who are subnormal may commit offences because of lack of understanding of the likely results of their behaviour, or because of exploitation by others. Sexual offences, especially indecent exposure, and arson, are the only offences closely associated with mental handicap. The rate of detection is higher in subnormal offenders than in those of normal intelligence.

Alcohol And Drug Abuse

There are a number of crimes which are specific to alcohol abuse, for example, being drunk and disorderly and driving under the influence of alcohol. However, in addition, crimes of violence are common due to the disinhibiting effect of alcohol coupled with an increase in irritability and querulousness. Though this may involve strangers, as in drunken public house brawls, not infrequently the victim is known to the offender, for example in cases of morbid jealousy. Crimes against property are also common, whether criminal damage committed when drunk or theft in order to obtain drink. Though alcohol and drugs may produce a state of intoxication in which the person is not fully aware of what he is doing, self-induced intoxication is no defence unless *a* the crime necessitates specific intent, for example, murder or theft, or *b* the intoxication is evidence of disease of the mind and therefore qualifies for the plea of not guilty by reason of insanity under the McNaughton rules. Finally alcohol abuse may lead to many different secondary psychiatric syndromes which may conduce to criminal activity; for example, paranoid psychoses.

Crimes may also be specific to drug abuse, for example, possession, making or marketing of illicit drugs; or they may be secondary to the pharmacological effects of the drugs, as in toxic psychoses with paranoid flavours, or they may be carried out in order to acquire money for drugs.

FAMILY LAW

The psychiatrist will be involved in this branch of law mainly as a result of custody hearings or more rarely in divorce or nullity petitions. In custody hearings the mental state of one or both parties will be relevant in so far as it affects child rearing. This includes the presence of psychiatric illness in the parent which is deleterious to the child, and a past or present history of child neglect or abuse.

CIVIL LAW

The psychiatrist may be called upon in post-injury compensation cases, accusations of medical negligence, or court protection orders.

Compensation issues

Psychiatrists are sometimes asked to give opinions on people who have been involved in accidents. This includes firstly assessing the degree of organic brain sequelae following head injuries, secondly commenting upon the presence of functional psychiatric symptomatology and its relationship to the accident, and thirdly commenting on the aetiology of any remaining physical symptoms for which no adequate organic cause can be found.

Organic sequelae after head injuries

These may be acute or chronic. Acute effects involve impairment of consciousness and amnesia for events surrounding the injury. The latter can be divided into retrograde amnesia — loss of memory for events leading up to the accident; and post-traumatic amnesia — which is defined as amnesia lasting from the moment of injury until the resumption of normal continuous memory. Retrograde amnesia is usually shorter than post-traumatic amnesia, shrinks with time as cerebral function returns, and is of much less diagnostic and prognostic significance. A close relationship exists betwen post-traumatic amnesia and the presence of permanent psychiatric disability and/or intellectual impairment.

The chronic sequelae are listed in Table 10.3. It must be remembered that although over half the patients who develop post-traumatic epilepsy do so within the first year and seventy-five per cent within four years, the risk of doing so still remains after that period of time, albeit at a decreased level. Post-traumatic epilepsy is most likely to occur after the dura mater has been pierced, in the presence of a depressed skull fracture or cranial haematoma, following a post-traumatic amnesia greater than twenty-four hours, and a fit in the first week after the injury. It may lead to intellectual and psychosocial disturbances.

Psychological sequelae

Psychiatric illness and personality disturbance may follow brain damage directly, when the symptoms are usually related to site and severity or to the later development of epilepsy; or they may be a reaction to the injury and its sequelae.

Post-traumatic neurosis

Post-traumatic neurosis may follow any injury regardless of site. Although usually seen as reactive to the accident, where is follows a head injury it may also be due to limbic brain damage. The symptoms of post-traumatic neurosis include depression, anxiety, irritability, fatigue and physical symptoms. The most important differential diagnosis is from malingering, usually for compensation purposes.

Malingering

The diagnosis of malingering depends on positive criteria which are:
1 The patient admits he is lying.
2 The patient is seen doing something which he says he is not able to do.
3 The patient's assertion of incapacity and incapability is manifestly at odds with the facts; for example, a man who says he cannot use his hands and yet without any outside help appears in the consulting room neatly dressed. Although malingering does occur it is rare in frequency when compared with post-traumatic neurosis.

Sexual dysfunction

Sexual difficulties are not uncommon after injury and may include loss of libido and impairment of arousal or orgasm. Though they may in some cases be organic and directly due to the injury (see Chapter 6), they are often psychological in nature.

Table 10.3 Chronic organic sequelae of head injuries

Intellectual impairment	Risk increases with age
Epilepsy	Most commonly temporal lobe epilepsy in closed head injuries
Personality change	Frontal lobe damage Temporal lobe damage Basal syndrome
Psychosis	Schizophrenia, related to site and severity of injury Paranoid psychosis ⎱ unrelated to site Affective psychosis ⎰ or severity of injury

Important factors include fear of damage, associated mood distrubance, performance anxiety following an initial period of sexual failure, and loss of self-esteem. This latter may be a direct consequence of the accident which expresses the vulnerability of the person and/or due to changes in general prowess consequent on the accident.

Aetiological factors in the development of post-traumatic psychiatric symptoms

Aetiological factors which determine the development of psychiatric problems following an accident include consitutional factors such as age, premorbid personality with the vulnerable and obsessionally rigid being most at risk, emotional effects of the accident and subsequent injury, environmental factors, site and amount of brain damage, consequent development of epilepsy and compensation issues.

Persistent physical symptoms

In a number of cases physical symptoms referrable to the site of the injury persist long after any organic damage has resolved. Psychologically, these symptoms may be aspects of conversion hysteria relating to the emotional trauma of the accident, somatic sympsions of anxiety, depressive equivalents or rarely, due to malingering. The diagnosis of physical symptoms due to psychological disorder is dealt with in Chapter 21.

MENTAL HEALTH ACT 1983

The minutiae of the Mental Health Act are outside the remit of this book, but it is, relevant to outline the psychiatric criteria for admission to hospital under the Mental Health Act 1983. The patient must be suffering from a mental disorder as defined by the Act and this includes mental illness, arrested or incomplete development of mind, and psychopathic disorder. The mental disorder must be of a nature or degree which warrants the detention of the patient in hospital: that is, if he were not so detained his own health or safety and/or the safety of others would be at risk. Promiscuity or other immoral conduct, sexual deviancy, or dependency on alcohol or drugs are by themselves

not sufficient criteria for the application of the Act. If the mental disorder is one of psychopathic disorder or mental impairment then in order to make an order under the Mental Health Act these conditions must be considered treatable.

CASE HISTORY

MR BOLT

Mr Bolt, a 31-year-old man, was remanded in custody on a charge of indecent assault of a minor, and a psychiatric opinion was sought. The charge involved three occasions on which Mr Bolt was said to have mutually masturbated three young boys between 11 and 13 years in age. They had been frequent visitors to his house and had consented to this sexual activity for which they had been given small presents. At no time had there been any violence or coercion. Mr Bolt had two previous offences for similar behaviour, the first of which had resulted in probation and the second in a short custodial sentence. There had been no other forensic history of either sexual or other criminal offences.

Mr Bolt was known to be a loner and in the five years since had had come to live on the estate he had made no friends. Word had got around about his previous offences and he had been ostracized by the local community. Although children had been discouraged from talking to Mr Bolt he had become known as a soft touch for money and presents. His only social outlet was the cinema, which he visisted on his own on a regular basis. His sole companion was his dog whom he looked after assiduously. While he was on probation attempts had been made to increase his social skills and opportunities, but he had shown little motivation to do so and had even had to be persuaded to bath regularly so that he did not smell.

He was born illegitimately and was initially brought up by his mother and grandparents. His grandfather drank heavily and often beat his mother and grandmother; and the atmosphere in the parental home was an unpleasant one. The mother had many boyfriends and would disappear from home for days on end. When he was five his grandfather became ill with lung cancer and died some months later, followed soon afterwards by his grandmother. His mother was no longer able or willing to look after him and he was taken into care. He spent the next few years in an orphanage, where he was known as a loner who withdrew from social contacts and was bullied by the older boys. He frequently wet the bed at night, and left to himself his personal hygiene was poor. At school he was noted as being lazy and sullen. His homework was rarely done and when it was, the quality was very poor. He had great difficulty in reading and writing and was barely numerate. He was no more successful on the sports field and none of the other children included him in their games. At the age of ten he was referred to an educational psychologist who performed tests of his intellectual ability. He was found to be educationally subnormal and was referred to a special school where he fared no better and frequently got into trouble for not trying. Once more he was picked on by his peers.

At the age of sixteen he left school with no qualifications. He obtained a job sweeping up in a factory where the isolation suited him but his timekeeping was poor as was the quality of his work, and within six months he was sacked. Since then had had been unable to find any regular employment.

He had always had difficulty making friends and been seen as a loner. He had never had any girlfriends and was shy in female company. He had had two brief homosexual relationships, one during his teens and one some five years later. Neither had lasted more than a few months and in both he had been the passive partner. He masturbated fairly regularly to fantasies involving the fondling of young boys, though buggery was never a part of the fantasy. There was no history of drug or alcohol abuse.

QUESTIONS

What are the aetiological factors behind Mr Bolt's sexual deviancy?
What is the prognosis in this case?

What recommendations should be made to the court as regards sentence?

Mr Bolt was brutally brought up in a household where he never saw a normal man-woman relationship and at an early age he was taken into care. He never found it easy to mix and never learned to socialize. It may thus have been that the company of young children was the only social outlet that he had and the only escape from a life of loneliness. His low IQ may also have contributed to his finding children easier to mix with. The history of homosexual reationships and fantasies suggests that his sexual orientation was in this direction and may explain the exact nature of his offences.

Given the history of two previous offences of a similar nature, without changes in his social circumstances it is difficult to see why he should not reoffend in the future. His low IQ and previously poor motivation make it unlikely that he will comply with or respond to treatment. Because of his difficulty in socializing it is unlikely that he will increase his social outlets to enable him to mix with adults rather than children. As far as his sexual orientation is concerned there is no reason or desire to expect that this will change and the aim would be for him to make relationships with adult men rather than young boys though his social deficiencies make this impracticable. His past history suggests that future offences will not involve violence but will be carried out with the implicit or explicit consent of the young boys involved.

As he is unlikely to respond to or comply with treatment there is no point in suggesting a medical recommendation of treatment. One may be able to give an answer on the risk of future offences but it is up to the legal authorities to determine whether a custodial sentence is appropriate and if so how long that should be. One difficulty in assessing motivation for treatment is that patients may protest that they will comply with any and all treatment suggested in order to avoid being locked up. One can only advise on previous knowledge of this patient and experience of similar people.

11

Disorders of speech

Normal speech patterns are difficult to define, since they are wide-ranging, both between and within individuals. A pragmatic definition is that speech is disordered when it fails to convey what the speaker intends, but this is a limited view since it does not account for variations in perception and comprehension in the listener. Speech is only one aspect of language, but its specific function is to communicate with others, although communication is also achieved by other methods.

This chapter will focus mainly on abnormalities of the form rather than the content of speech. The latter will only be described here where it severely affects communication, but will be dealt with in more detail in Chapter 12 (Disorders of Thinking).

It is important to establish whether a patient with a speech disorder is functioning at his own optimum level, or whether his speech has deteriorated after normal development in childhood. Distinction into primary and secondary disorder is important in diagnosis.

PRIMARY SPEECH DISORDER (Table 11.1)

Speech begins to develop at around one year of age, and most children are using phrases or sentences by the age of two. Development is considered delayed if speech is not present by the age of three or three-and-a-half years. Normal speech depends on normal development of the respiratory system in addition to central nervous system maturation and intact hearing.

Speech distortions or *dysarthria* may occur as a result of neuromuscular disorders, cleft palate, or hearing impairment. Such distortions may be

Table 11.1 Primary speech disturbance

Distortions (dysarthria)	Neuromuscular disorders Local pathology e.g. cleft palate Hearing impairment
Failure to acquire speech	Deafness Lack of stimulus Mental handicap Infantile autism Developmental dysphasia

completely overcome by a combination of medical treatment and education, but may also persist throughout life, rendering verbal communication more difficult. Speech form should not be affected in these conditions, although some congenitally profoundly deaf individuals never achieve adequate speech and will use a combination of a few words and many gestures to communicate.

Failure to acquire adequate speech may be secondary to deafness or lack of stimulus, or may be a feature of a generalized mental subnormality or of early childhood psychosis. It may also occur as a primary language deficit — *developmental dysphasia* — and may occur with developmental dyslexia and dysgraphia. Developmental dysphasia may result from birth trauma and may be associated with other signs of cerebral palsy. The greater plasticity of the infantile cerebrum frequently allows the right hemisphere to become dominant if the left is damaged at birth, but this process is often incomplete, leading to delay in language milestones. Language function may be globally affected but most commonly expressive language is defective and comprehension is unimpaired. Receptive dysphasia may be difficult to distinguish from deafness and may be associated with it. Although neurological signs are often absent in cases of development dysphasia, most authorities consider it to be of organic origin. However, the site of the causative lesion remains unknown, although it may be in parietal association areas.

Children with severe receptive and expressive developmental dysphasia may appear mentally handicapped and it is essential to distinguish between specific language disorders and those cases where speech failure reflects a general cerebral disorder. Psychomotor testing must be thorough, and repeated as the child develops, in order for the diagnosis to be reliable. Early infantile autism invariably involves language function, so that comprehension and communication, both verbal and non-verbal, are severely affected. Many autistic children are mute, and in those who do speak, repetitive, stereotyped and idiosyncratic patterns develop so that the speech is incomprehensible unless interpreted by someone who knows the child well. The diagnosis of infantile autism depends on identifying impairment of social interaction, imaginative play, and repetitive activity in addition to language failure.

Speech will not develop unless the child hears speech, so that seriously disrupted parents who neither play with their children, nor speak to them or to each other, and who are socially isolated, will produce children whose speech is delayed and impoverished. Speech delay in these circumstances reflects the emotional impact of severe deprivation, as well as the lack of opportunity to learn the significance of speech.

The assessment of a language-impaired child depends not only on the paediatrician and neurologist, but on a team including educational psychologist, audiologist and speech therapist, and in some cases a child psychiatrist.

SECONDARY SPEECH DISTURBANCES
(Table 11.2)

Deterioration in verbal ability, after it has initially been achieved, occurs from neurological and psychiatric causes. The assessment of speech disorders must take account of the many variables which affect speech. Intelligence, education,

Table 11.2 Secondary speech disturbance

Rate	Retarded
	Increased
Quantity	Reduced
	Increased
Flow	Dysarthria
	Stammering, Stuttering
	Mutism
	Aphonia
	Aphasia
Content	Mannerism
	Stereotypies — verbigeration
	Schizophrenic thought disorder
	including: schizophasia
	neologisms
	echolalia
	Perseveration
	Coprolalia
	Talking past the point(*vorbeireden*)
	Flight of ideas

culture, and personality all contribute to the way an individual habitually uses words. Whether the language spoken is native to the patient or learnt in adulthood may also be important. Speech is also dependent on the prevailing psychological state; anxiety, unhappiness and excitement may change the rate, flow and coherence of speech to a marked degree. Some patients may be rendered speechless by the stress of attending surgery or the hospital, and this must be taken into account.

The assessment of speech as part of the wider examination of the mental state of the patient is important, not only to identify major abnormalities, but also to note variations in speech pattern which add to the picture of each individual patient. Where speech is overtly abnormal, samples should be recorded verbatim for later analysis, since doctors differ in their understanding of some of the terms used in the assessment and description of speech. It is important to judge whether verbal fluency is congruent with the educational attainments and occupation of the patient, or whether the manner of his speech portrays his mood.

Rate of speech

The pace of speech may markedly be altered in

affective states. Severely depressed people may show a retardation in speech and movement so that responses are delayed and slow, whereas hypomanic or excited patients will talk rapidly and at length, and ignore the non-verbal cues which normally indicate that a pause and switch in dialogue is appropriate. Such rapid flow, termed pressure of speech, may occur in schizophrenics and in anxious people. As hypomania becomes more severe, the communicative function of speech is disrupted, so that the patient verbalizes, uncensored, the multiplicity of racing thoughts which crowd his mind.

Flight of ideas

Flight of ideas is the term given to speech in which the content appears to jump from topic to topic, but on closer observation can be seen to contain connections between the themes. These links may be of content, when it appears as if the missing connecting thread has been omitted, probably because the patient is thinking faster than he can talk; alternatively, the links may be via sounds, as in clanging or rhyming speech, or via words, as in puns. Flight of ideas occurs in mania and is usually associated with pressure of speech. It should not be confused with schizophrenic thinking, where the patient may also jump from topic to topic but where there are no connections between them and there is no pressure of speech. An example of flight of ideas is, 'I'm going down the road to see Mrs Bird, cheep cheep, soap powder's very cheap today . . . .'

Quantity of speech

Too little speech, so that the individual talks in monosyllables or short phrases and includes insufficient detail without prompting by the interviewer, may be caused by anxiety, and the amount of speech may vary through the interview as topics which cause greater or less tension are encountered. It may also convey hostility, in patients who are reluctant to be interviewed; suggest preoccupation with the internal world; reflect low intelligence; or be a longstanding feature of personality in patients who are shy and lack social skills. Depressed, retarded patients also show poverty of speech, and schizophrenic patients preoccupied by their voices may be otherwise engaged.

Over production of speech, so that the patient talks at length, but at a normal pace, may be a personality variable in people who are gregarious and expansive, but may also denote anxiety. Some patients will talk excessively on some topics to avoid thinking about other painful areas, and one has to be alert to this form of evasion. Patients with obsessional personalities often talk at length, particularly in a situation such as a medical examination, in their need to be quite sure that they have conveyed all relevant details of their history, together with exact dates of all variations in their symptoms. Talking too much may simply reflect loneliness, or lack of experience in social interaction.

Excessive speech may fall into distinct patterns. It may be entirely to the point, but inappropriately detailed, as in the obsessional patient, or it may be *circumstantial* in that the general theme of the conversation is maintained, but the patient repeatedly digresses on to a related topic for a while before returning to the matter in hand. *Discursive* speech occurs when the train of thought is not maintained but each topic is exhaustively discussed before another is embarked on. *Over-inclusion* is an aspect of schizophrenic thought disorder and its occurrence in speech must be differentiated from circumstantiality. Speech which is over-inclusive contains elements which are irrelevant to the main direction of the speech, but which are held by the speaker to be central to the topic. The patient cannot focus on the topic in hand because he has a distorted view of the limits of the subject. For example, if a circumstantial patient describing the onset of her back pain digresses to the detail of the weather and what her neighbour at the bus stop said, the day the pain began, she will realize she has digressed when prompted by a question which brings her back to the pain. A schizophrenic patient will show over-inclusion when he describes all the thoughts associated with a particular event and will be bewildered that the interviewer is not enlightened by his detail. Over-inclusion always occurs with other aspects of thought disorder in schizophrenia (see chapter 12).

Flow

Dysarthria, where the mechanical production of speech is impaired as in bulbar palsy, causes alterations in flow.

Stammering occurs when the flow of speech is arrested by pauses and repetition of parts of words. Stuttering is often used synonymously although some authorities use this term to refer to a more severe stammer. Its frequency is highest in children, where its peak ages of onset are at two to three and six to eight years, but it may persist into adulthood or recur in adulthood at times of stress. Stammering rarely begins after puberty. It is much commoner and tends to persist longer in boys. Stammering most often affects the beginning of words, and may be accompanied by grimaces or gestures. Speaking quickly, and anxiety, tend to worsen the condition but other emotional states such as anger may improve it, as does singing or speaking in unison. Its aetiology remains a subject of debate but psychological factors are undoubtedly involved in many cases. There is a familial tendency to stammer and some evidence that it is commoner in monozygotic twins and in those with incomplete cerebral dominance for language. Stammering can be altered by interfering with auditory feedback; whether its dependence on auditory perception of the voice is entirely physiological or also psychological remains unclear.

Mutism

Mutism is defined as complete loss of speech and may be due to psychiatric or neurological disorders. Mutism in children who have achieved speech is usually elective in that they will speak in some situations and with some people, but not in others. It usually signifies serious emotional disturbance, but may be evidence of a developing psychotic illness. Mutism occurs in the stupor of catatonic schizophrenia and severe depressive illness, although in the latter some attempt may be made to speak. Stuporose patients are immobile in addition to being silent, and will have other neurological signs, if the disorder is of organic origin, as in akinetic mutism. Other schizophrenic patients may be silent for delusional reasons, for

instance obeying alien forces forbidding them to communicate. Mutism is an effective way of exhibiting anger, and may reflect deliberate non-cooperation. *Aphonia*, rather than mutism, occurs as a conversion in hysteria; when faced with overwhelming stress, the patient converts his anxiety into a physical symptom. In aphonia, the words are mouthed or whispered, but the larynx is not involved in word production. However, the diagnosis becomes clear on demonstration of normal coughing which shows that the larynx is functionally intact. As would be expected, non-verbal communication is unaffected. Some schizophrenics may only speak in a whisper, either as a mannerism or in response to delusions or hallucinations. *Aphasia* is the complete loss, *dysphasia* the partial loss, of comprehension and/or expression of speech resulting from a lesion in the language area of the dominant cerebral hemisphere. The commonest cause is a cerebrovascular accident, but any focal intracerebral pathology, such as neoplasm, abscess or trauma may be responsible. Aphasia will develop in dementia when the language area becomes affected by the general cortical decay; but failure of cognition and memory may supervene in the clinical picture, so that the classic forms of aphasia are no longer identifiable.

Aphasia can be classified as expressive when language is comprehended but cannot be formulated, or receptive, when the understanding of speech is impaired. Expressive dysphasia is caused by a lesion in Broca's area (the posterior part of the inferior frontal convolution), receptive dysphasia by a lesion in the posterior part of the superior temporal gyrus. Central aphasia results in difficulty in comprehension and expression in both spoken and written language.

Dysphasias are also described as fluent (posterior lesions) or non-fluent (anterior lesions). Fluent dysphasias are those where cadence and flow of speech is normal, but affected individuals speak more and are often incoherent due to abnormal sounds and neologisms. Fluent dysphasia involving both understanding and expression is called Wernicke's aphasia. Non-fluent dysphasia is predominantly motor and speech output is severely or completely reduced. Only a few words or phrases may be uttered, and syntax and rhythm are always impaired. Perseveration (see below) also occurs. Nominal aphasia is a type of non-fluent dysphasia where the predominant sign is difficulty in naming objects, together with impaired fluency in ordinary speech.

Aphasia is often associated with some impairment in reading (dyslexia), writing (dysgraphia), use of objects (apraxia) and recognition (agnosia). Since comprehensive neurological examination is mandatory in all cases of acquired impairment of language there should be no difficulty in recognizing the organic nature of the dysphasias. However, early, minor, or atypical lesions may cause some initial confusion over diagnosis, especially in patients with previous or current psychiatric history or an unusually marked variation in speech ability according to the prevailing emotional state.

Disorders of speech content

Since speech reflects thought, abnormalities of content are most logically considered in the chapters on disorders of thought and abnormal ideation. Nevertheless, in certain situations, disorders of speech form render the content of speech so disturbed as to become incomprehensible.

Mannerisms and stereotypes

Verbal mannerisms of intonation, pronunciation and other aspects of speech production are found in catatonia. Where speech is punctuated by constant repetition of specific words and phrases out of context, this is called verbal stereotypy. This is also found in catatonia and may occur in mental handicap and organic brain disease. Speech consisting of continual stereotypies is called verbigeration.

Gross examples of catatonic speech disorder, although common in the early descriptions of the condition, are now rarely found in Western psychiatric practice. Schizophrenic patients may show a lesser degree of speech disorder in that their utterances are normally comprehensible despite some peculiarities of syntax, but with evidence that some 'stock' words are used in an especial and privately symbolic way. *Neologisms* are newly constructed words which are similarly

used in a way which indicates they have a special meaning for the patient, and also occur in organic disorders.

Occasionally in schizophrenia, disorder of thought form may render speech totally incomprehensible. This nonsense speech is known as schizophasia, speech confusion or word salad.

Echolalia

Echolalia occurs when the patient repeats the whole or part of what has been said to him. It is a stage in childhood babble, and its occurrence in advanced dementia as well as catatonic schizophrenia is indicative of a loss of acquired language skills and a return to a primitive level of function.

Perseveration

Perseveration is a disorder of speech which is distinguished from stereotyped utterance by the fact that its timing is understandable. For example a perseverative patient may answer 'October' to an enquiry about the month of the year and continue to say 'October' when asked the year, the day of the week and so on. Although perseveration may occur in schizophrenia its presence is usually a mark of organic deterioration and may be an early sign of developing dementia. Consequently organic disease must always be considered in patients with this symptom, until it can be excluded.

Coprolalia

Coprolalia means explosive outbursts of foul speech, and is found in the syndrome of Gilles de la Tourette, where it is accompanied by grunting and abnormal movements.

Vorbeireden

In *vorbeireden*, or talking past the point, the patient may appear constantly on the verge of answering the question, or getting to the heart of the matter, but never achieves this. It is referred to in the Ganser syndrome, when the patient is thought deliberately to be giving answers which are inaccurate, but approximate to the topic. In this syndrome, the patient understands the question, but when talking past the point occurs in chronic schizophrenia, the patient is likely to be trying to discuss the topic to the best of his ability.

CASE HISTORY

ALYSHA BEGUM

Alysha Begum, a 25-year-old married woman originally from Bangladesh, was seen at home at her general practitioner's request. Her husband had visited the GP and said that he was worried about his wife who was not speaking, and was behaving oddly. She had been sitting in the bath pouring cold water over her head, had not been cooking or looking after the family, and had not seemed to know where she was or what she was doing. Her husband said that she had been totally uncommunicative with him, their children and other relatives, but would sometimes wail, and recite verses from the Koran. Her GP said that ten days earlier the couple's eldest son, aged nine, had been knocked down by a car a few yards from their home and was in intensive care; permanent brain damage was suspected.

Although her husband's English was good, Alysha Begum's was not, and so an independent interpreter accompanied the psychiatrist on the assessment. Alysha was found sitting on the floor, rocking, rubbing her hands over her head and pulling her sari over her face. She showed neither surprise nor emotion at the visit, and could not be persuaded to say anything at all. Her husband was agitated and upset, and showed the psychiatrist burnt saucepans, perishable food put in cupboards and not the fridge, and a towel torn into strips, as evidence of his wife's unnatural behaviour — she was normally an exemplary housewife. When Alysha was questioned about these things and about the fact that her husband said she had been sitting in a bath of cold water for hours the previous night, she clearly understood what she was being asked, gave a faint shrug, but otherwise said nothing. She had two other children, aged five and three years, neither of whom could engage her attention.

Alysha was reported as having been very calm when her neighbour ran in to tell her that her son had been injured; she did not break down in tears until he was admitted to hospital. She had sat by his bed wailing, and the nurses had asked her if she could be a little quieter. Her husband had been angry with her for not controlling herself and had taken her home. After her next visit to the hospital she had broken away from her husband and walked home alone — this was unheard-of in their family and was the first sign of abnormal behaviour. He had not thought it safe to allow her to visit her son subsequently; he spent much time at the bedside but did not tell his wife any details of his son's progress for fear of its effect on her mental state.

The couple had been married for ten years and had spent much of their early marriage apart whilst they awaited permission for Alysha to join her husband in England. He had been in England with his father since the age of twelve, twenty years before, and had returned to Bangladesh for his arranged marriage. Alysha had no significant past medical or psychiatric history, although she had been unhappy and prone to frequent minor illness during the first couple of years in England. None of her family was in England, and she had been very sad and withdrawn for a while the previous year when she heard of her maternal grandmother's death.

Her husband claimed that they got on well together, and had no problems apart from their anxiety about their son's accident. He did not think that her current state could be explained by anxiety; he thought that she was mentally ill, needed looking after and was not safe to be left at home, especially with the care of their younger children. He requested that she be admitted to hospital.

Questions

What is the likely differential diagnosis?
What further steps should be taken to establish it?
What particular difficultieis of transcultural work does this case illustrate?

It is premature to give a differential diagnosis at this stage, since much more information is required, but an initial plan of management is needed now, so some diagnostic possibilities must be explored. It is apparent that Begum Alysha's changed mental state is related to her son's accident, but whether her reaction to this is culturally normal or not is uncertain, particularly in the face of her husband's contention that it is not. Her muteness may be evidence of a depressive or catatonic stupor, but there is no other evidence in her mental state to support either diagnosis. She is in touch with her surroundings, although unreactive to them. Her muteness is apparently not selective; she is not talking to anyone. It is not specifically directed at her husband.

Her unreliability at her household tasks may mean that she is too preoccupied or too anxious, that she cannot concentrate or that she does not think these things are important at present. At this stage, it could be for any or all of these reasons, and it certainly is premature to attribute any strong psychiatric significance to this complaint.

At first sight, her bathing does seem abnormal, but on discussion with the interpreter (who was from the same culture) it became clear that Alysha was performing Islamic cleansing rituals, albeit to somewhat excessive extent.

The most likely diagnosis is that this is a traumatic reaction in a woman made vulnerable by distance from a supportive family, and living in an alien culture, whose language she does not understand. A hysterical dissociation is a probability, although there is no evidence of a previous hysterical tendency. It is also possible that she is wilfully mute, and behaving in a consciously bizarre fashion, for reasons which are not, as yet, clear. It is unlikely that she has a psychotic illness.

The next stage in assessment is to establish whether Alysha can be persuaded to talk to anybody. She would be most likely to seek, and derive, support from female relatives, were she at home, and so it is important to find out if she has any sisters-in-law, or whether her relationship with her mother-in-law is a good one. It is also important to remember that she may be uneasy about talking to a male psychiatrist; under these circumstances the opportunity for her to see the interpreter alone may be valued.

Perhaps the most useful next step, however, would be to arrange for Alysha to visit her son in hospital; preferably with someone she trusts other than her husband, and preferably with the support and encouragement of the nursing staff in the intensive care unit. Her anxiety may be helped by seeing him; her expressions of grief may be facilitated and not misunderstood as they were on the previous occasion. If, however, she does not improve as a result, this may be evidence for the existence of mental illness.

This case illustrates problems of transcultural psychiatry in assessing the significance of altered, but not severely bizarre, behaviour in people with different lifestyles and customs. In addition, where language is a barrier, it is also difficult to assess mental state, and essential to have an independent interpreter.

Alysha began to speak in front of her sister-in-law, with whom she visited her son, and it became clear that she was angry with her husband for his failure to support her through her anxiety about her son's accident, for which she felt guilty. This was because she had given him permission to go out and buy some sweets, after her husband had previously refused; it was on her son's return from the sweetshop that his accident occurred. She had not told her husband of this, and it would not have been easy to elicit this information if he had been interpreting for her.

The other major problem in assessing this situation is how much one should react to her husband's anxiety and belief in his wife's mental illness as strong evidence in favour of a psychiatric diagnosis. Certainly, if he believes the situation is not understandable in terms of her previous personality and culture it is difficult for those not of her culture to reject this as evidence. However, it may be, as transpired in this case, that his difficulty was that he had never been previously called upon to share and support a grieving, anxious woman, and did not understand the form that such distress took. In their country of origin, in the presence of a large extended family, Alysha would have depended largely on her female relatives, and might not have turned to him for much emotional support.

12

Disorders of thinking

Disturbances in thought processes occur in many psychiatric diseases and it is important to develop the skill of identifying and describing those abnormalities which are of diagnostic significance. In the mental state examination, thought and speech function should be considered separately although thought disorders will be identified by the interviewer via the speech pattern of the patient. To some extent, speech allows the objective study of parts of the subjective experience of thought.

NORMAL THINKING

Normal thinking is directed in two main areas; the inner life of the individual, which is a complex blend of thoughts, feelings and images which may not be constructed into verbal language, and the interacting part of the self which formulates thoughts with a view to action, speech, decisions and so on. Apart from the use of 'thinking' as equivalent to 'believing' in European languages, there are three types of thinking which form part of everyday individual mental life.

Conceptual thinking

Conceptual thinking is reality-based, more or less logical, and goal-directed. Much of ordinary daily activity and working life is taken up with rational, problem-solving thinking. Intelligence is an important factor in its successful function and personality traits account for variations in the amount of energy and time people devote to this type of thinking. Traits such as punctiliousness, perfectionism, ambition and a high drive towards achievement tend to be associated with a high

degree of conceptual thinking. Variations of mood affect rational thinking and can disrupt it completely. Loss of interest in life, as in depression, may render problem-solving pointless, and the loss of concentration which is also a feature of depression may relate to the loss of the ability to think through a rational sequence. Excitement and overactivity will also disrupt the smooth conceptual process.

Imaginative thinking

This type of thinking is fundamentally creative. It also is goal-directed and has logical elements, but it moves somewhat beyond the bounds of rationality and reality. It is abstract, inventive and an essential part of the development of human culture, both artistically and technologically. The individual variation in imaginative ability is again wide, and at the extreme produces great writers, composers and scientists.

Dereistic thinking

This term was coined by Bleuler to describe non-goal-directed, wish-fulfilling thinking. It is purely fantasy and recognized in popular language as daydreaming. It is a normal aspect of thinking which can refresh and enrich mental life and it may connect with the other types of thought in its contrast and clarification of them. For instance, extended periods of dereistic thinking seem to be important in adolescence as a melting pot for the development of ego ideals and of aims and objectives for adult life. It is characteristically increased during other transitions such as marriage, parenthood and bereavement, and has an important function as a comfort in times of stress and loneliness. It is abnormal when it is excessive or inappropriately timed and indicates neurotic and intrapersonal problems when it is consistently indulged in at the cost of other activities. Dereistic thinking should always be recognized as fantasy by the individual; the blurring of this boundary is pathological and indicates the development of a psychotic illness.

Abnormalities of thought

The examination of thought pathology must include four main areas: difficulties in thought stream, thought content, thought possession and thought form. Since disorders of the stream of thought are largely considered in the chapter on speech disorders, and thought content in chapter 17 on abnormal beliefs, the greater part of this chapter will concentrate on disorders of possession and form.

DISORDERS OF THOUGHT POSSESSION

Thought alienation

Thought alienation is the experience that all or part of one's thoughts are not one's own, or that one has no control over them. There are three forms of thought alienation: broadcasting, insertion and withdrawal. They all occur in acute schizophrenia and are, in the absence of organic brain disease, virtually diagnostic of it. They are all classified by Schneider as first rank symptoms for the diagnosis of schizophrenia, and their presence indicated a probability of over 90% of diagnosis of schizophrenia in the WHO International Study of Schizophrenia. Evidence of thought alienation, therefore, must be elicited with care, partly because it is easy to misunderstand the patient's description of his experience and identify it as present when it is not. It is important to have verbatim descriptions from the patient, and to question the original statements, in order to avoid false positive responses.

Thought broadcasting

Thought broadcasting is the experience that one's own thoughts can be placed in other people's minds. It is not the same as the belief that one's thoughts can be read, but is rather a belief that one's thoughts are shared by others in unison. An example of thought broadcasting is the statement, 'I don't have to tell you what I am thinking because you're thinking my thoughts'. It must be distinguished from the occurrence of the same ideas to different people at the same time — 'two minds with a single thought' — by the fact that the experience of thought broadcasting contains the essential element that it is *my* thoughts which are in *your* head, not just that the thoughts are coincidental but independent of each other. There is also a concrete quality to this phenomenon as if the thoughts have physically travelled from the patient's brain to that of the onlooker.

Thought insertion

Thought insertion is the experience of thoughts being placed inside the patient's mind, so that he recognizes that some or all of his thoughts are not his own, are not under his control, and are nothing to do with him. It is essential to establish that the patient actually experiences the thoughts as foreign. Patients with thought insertion will usually have a belief about the origin of the thoughts — for example, the thoughts are placed there by lasers, computers, or particular people who are controlling him. A common mistake in the examination of this symptom is to interpret statements such as, 'I don't know why I think that — that's not me at all' as thought insertion. This occurs because of a misinterpretation by the examiner of the tendency to disown unpleasant, dangerous or shameful thoughts by saying, 'It's not (like) me to think these things'. The difference between 'I'd rather not have these thoughts' and 'I really know these thoughts aren't mine' can be established by asking a further question such as, '*How* can you — anyone — have thoughts in your head which are nothing to do with you?' Only patients whose ability to distinguish their self from the outside world is impaired will respond by a positive description of an insertion; patients with other conditions where the integrity of the self is preserved will give an answer such as, 'Well of course they *must* be mine — can't be anyone else's — I suppose I mean what sort of person am I to have such ideas'.

Thought withdrawal

Thought withdrawal is the experience of thoughts being removed from one's head, sometimes again with elaborate beliefs about the mechanism. Some patients experience the thoughts as being removed through a particular route, for example, the ear or the top of the head, and will find their minds a partial or total blank. Again, it is important to identify the experience of *removal* and not just the resulting blankness.

Thought blocking

Thought blocking is the experience of thoughts 'going blank' and its occurrence may denote thought withdrawal, although this cannot be assumed without direct evidence. Thought withdrawal is only one of the causes of blocking, which, as an interruption of thought continuity, is classified under disorders of thought stream. Blocking occurs in normal people who are fatigued or anxious about marshalling their thoughts for, say, a public meeting, and it also occurs in the absences of petit mal. If blocking is complained of by the patient, it is essential to ask, 'What happens to your thoughts; where/how do they go?' before thought withdrawal can be either demonstrated or discounted.

Obsessions

An obsession is defined as recurrent thought or image which arises unbidden to the mind, and against the will of the individual. Such thoughts are resisted but the individual cannot drive them from his mind without experiencing unbearable anxiety. The thoughts or images are repeated, sometimes continuously (obsessional ruminations), and may give rise to compulsive acts or rituals. Compulsions do not arise without obsessional thoughts, but thoughts may be present without compulsion. This is a neurotic, not a psychotic symptom, and the patient remains aware that he owns the thoughts, however unpleasant that awareness may be. On occasion it is diffucult to distinguish obsessional thinking from thought insertion, especially if the patient uses vivid imagery to describe it: 'It's the Devil putting all these dreadful thoughts into my mind'; but close questioning will reveal that the patient does not disown the origin of the thought but is saying, 'It's *as if* the Devil . . .'

In addition, the phenomenon itself should aid identification in that obsessions are frequently sexual, aggressive or obscene in content and the quality of repetition despite resistance, and inability to stop, is a pattern quite specific to this symptom.

Obsessions occur as transient non-disabling phenomena in patients of obsessional personality; as severe disabling symptoms in obsessive-compulsive neurosis and in depressive illness. They may occur in schizophrenia or in chronic organic psychosis, but have no diagnostic significance in either case. The differential diagnosis of the underlying conditions depends on other features of the history and mental state.

DISORDERS OF THOUGHT FORM

Under this heading are considered problems in the construction of language. Hence grammar, syntax and the appropriate use of words are the functions involved. In the early stages of disordered thought form, patients may complain of a difficulty in thought construction and talk in a vague, woolly fashion which is difficult to follow. Examination of verbatim speech reveals that subjects and objects are misplaced, that verbs and pronouns may be missing, so that the meaning of the speech may be difficult to understand. Patients with thought disorder may be perplexed and bewildered and struggle to make themselves comprehensible.

Disorders of thought form are found in organic brain disease and schizophrenia. Minor grammatical anomalies are not considered pathological if they are appropriate to the intelligence and education of the patient. *Acute organic states* produce abnormal thinking patterns, principally because consciousness, and hence alertness, is impaired and thoughts are interrupted. *Dementia*, where there is a global deterioration of cerebral function, causes these disorders as vocabulary is increasingly diminished and grammatical and syntactical rules of language construction are forgotten. The main diagnostic entity, however, in disorders of thought form, is schizophrenia. Some authorities use the terms 'schizophrenic thought disorder', 'formal thought disorder' and 'disorders of thought form' synonymously. The early descriptive literature on the clinical aspect of schizophrenia leans heavily towards this disorder and some authorities still consider schizophrenia as primarily a disorder of language. There is a large literature on the experimental investigation of schizophrenic language and the extent of its divergence from normal thought, details of which will not be considered here.

Schizophrenic thought disorder

Table 12.1 lists the classification of thought disorder as proposed by some authorities. It can be seen that there are many similarities between those concepts although they differ in their emphasis and their detail.

Bleuler considered schizophrenia to be primarily a disorder of association in that connections between ideas are disrupted, leading to variable and poorly differentiated concepts. He described three patterns of abnormality: *condensation*, *displacement*, and *misuse of symbols*. These terms were originally used by Freud in his analysis of the primary process thinking which characterizes dreams, and Bleuler used them in the same way. Condensation occurs when ideas with certain similarities are blended together to produce abnormal concepts; displacement is the substitution of one idea for a related one; and misuse of symbols is the use of words without their symbolic meaning. *Concrete thinking*, which is present when words are

used entirely without symbolic meaning, occurs in both organic states and schizophrenia, although whether the aetiology is the same in these conditions is disputed. Patients who demonstrate concrete thinking are unable to generalize concepts from specific examples; when asked to give the meaning of proverbs, for example, they will be unable to convey an understanding of the underlying principles. 'People who live in glass houses shouldn't throw stones' may be explained as 'Glass windows break when you throw things'. Since proverbs are particularly culture- and education-bound, it may be preferable to use the explanation of differences as a test for concrete thinking. For example, 'What's the difference between a car and a bus?' may produce a response such as, 'A car is black or blue and a bus is red'. Other workers have stressed the overinclusiveness of formal thought disorder, where boundaries between concepts are not maintained, and personal idiosyncratic themes are interpolated. Poor association of thoughts so that unrelated ideas are uttered in the course of an attempt to think along one train of thought is known as *tangential* or *knight's move* thinking. A knight in chess moves forward both vertically and diagonally, thus diverging from the original path. Thoughts which are largely tangential lead to speech which is incoherent.

In Schneider's classification, knight's move or *derailed* thinking occurs together with substitutions and omissions to form *transitory* thinking. *Drivelling* thinking is a failure of organization of thought so that a logical sequence is lost — this is akin to the concept of failure of association.

Table 12.1 Some Classification systems for thought disorder — showing similarities between them

Clinically	Bleuler	Cameron	Payne	Schneider
Loose, over-inclusive abnormalities of grammar and syntax	Disorder of association		Overinclusive	Drivelling thinking
	Condensation	Asyndesis		
Knight's move thinking	Displacement	Metonyms		Transitory thinking { derailment substitution omission
Concrete thinking	Misuse of symbols			
Introduction of unrelated concepts		Interpenetration of personal themes		Desultory thinking

Desultory thinking is defined as more or less normal in syntax but with the addition of new ideas unrelated to the topic in hand; this definition has similarities to concepts of overinclusion and interpenetration of themes.

Schizophrenic thought disorder is easier to recognize in a clinical setting that to understand from reading. It is an example of a clinical sign which once seen is never forgotten. For example, in the course of a lengthy attempt to explain why he found cities oppressive and uncongenial, a patient said, 'A house is not a bell because it's not built the same' and 'When you put curtains at the window a house dies'. Both these phrases, whilst conveying some kind of meaning, demonstrate overinclusiveness, and a faulty association of ideas. The first one is also an example of concrete thinking; whilst strictly true, it fails to convey the essential differences between houses and bells.

CASE HISTORY

ALAN GREEN

Alan, an unmarried man of 29, was referred for a psychiatric opinion, complaining that the Devil had entered into him, causing him to be wicked and sinful. He believed this to be the case because he had terrible thoughts of harm coming to his family, or indeed anyone about whom he cared. He pictured, in his mind, traumatic scenes in which loved ones were injured and mutilated, and also had thoughts of their being prevented from achieving a state of peace in the afterlife. Since he thought that he was, by nature, a peaceable and loving man, he could only understand the presence of these appalling thoughts if they had been caused by the Devil.

The thoughts began nine years before, and had changed only in detail and in emphasis during that time — their quality remained much the same. He had received various diagnoses and different treatment approaches but his condition had gradually worsened. Over the last few weeks, however, Alan had become more and more preoccupied with the ideas of harm in the afterlife, which distressed him even more than the thoughts of actual physical injury, since he was also plagued by the idea that he would never know what harm he had done or was doing to people who were dead, and hence could not tell him. He was, at present, completely preoccupied with these thoughts, which he described as going round and round in his head, causing him anxiety verging on panic, but which he could not prevent, however much he resisted the impulse to brood upon his ideas.

Some years before, he had first had the feeling that he might protect his family from damage if he carried out certain acts as a kind of expiation — he knew that this feeling was irrational, but having had this idea, he had to carry out the acts, just in case that would protect them; or, even worse, in case not doing them should expose his family to even more danger. These acts varied, but usually involved some sort of counting ritual, associated with everyday activities. For example, Alan had the compulsion to count to five before putting on his socks in the morning, and then to put his left sock on first — he also had to count to one hundred before crossing the threshold from one room to another. At first, these rituals had helped relieve his worry and doubt and had comforted him; however, within a few months, he began to doubt the accuracy of his counting, so that on reaching the target figure of, say, one hundred, he would not be sure that he had not made a mistake and *really* counted to one hundred and one or ninety-nine; so he would feel compelled to start again. Increasingly, he doubted whether he had ever got the correct number, so that he spent hours on end vacillating between one room and another, putting his clothes on, re-arranging the objects in his room, and so on.

It was only in the last two years that Alan had begun to explain his torment as being of satanic inspiration; he had come to this conclusion after long periods of introspection to find out whether he was as wicked as he felt.

There was no evidence of depression in his mental state, and there was no alteration of his sleep pattern, or loss of appetite or weight. Alan's family history was apparently unremarkable. His family were highly religious and both his parents attended church regularly and frequently. As a child he was extremely shy and made no friends at school, preferring to go train-spotting on his own, meticulously entering the numbers in a little book.

At the age of 18, he left home to study at university. He began a relationship with a girl, who was similarly shy, and this continued into his second year. This was his first relationship, and Alan felt inadequate and embarrassed about his sexual performance — no intercourse took place. The relationship ended when his girlfriend completed her course and returned to her home town; Alan was undecided about committing himself to her although he knew that she would have stayed if he had asked her to. On the break-up of the relationship, Alan became increasingly lonely and withdrawn, failed his second-year examinations, and in the ensuing long vacation at home he first developed the symptoms described above. He did not return to university, and apart from a few months working for a local solicitor, had neither worked, nor lived away from home, since. He was now a virtual recluse, with no contact with anyone outside his immediate family.

Questions

What is the likely differential diagnosis?
What particular features of his mental state are relevant to a solution to the diagnostic confusion?

The diagnosis of Alan's condition is either a severe obsessive-compulsive neurosis, or paranoid schizophrenia. Most of the phenomenology of Alan's complaints of rumination and ritualized behaviour is obsessional in nature. The symptoms are repetitive, and strongly resisted despite marked anxiety. This would suggest the diagnosis of obsessive compulsive neurosis. However, the principal issue is whether his belief that the Devil has caused this is delusional or not. If it is, then it is a delusion of passivity, a first rank symptom of schizophrenia, and the diagnosis is, most probably, one of paranoid schizophrenia. Even if Alan recognizes *some* of the symptoms as his own, true obsessional phenomena may occur in schizophrenia, although they are not of diagnostic significance.

There is no family history of schizophrenia, but Alan's premorbid personality would be compatible with the diagnosis. The onset of his deterioration is also quite common: the insidious development during late adolescence and declaration during times of stress is a frequent picture in schizophrenia.

The clue to the further elucidation of the symptom of being under the influence of the Devil is the assessment of the presence or absence of an 'as if' quality. If Alan is saying, in effect, 'I can find no way of accounting for the way my mind produces such dreadful thoughts other than by attributing them to the Devil — although I know that the thoughts must really be mine — it's as if the Devil were inside me', then this is compatible with an obsessional neurosis. If, however, he is saying, 'These thoughts are completely foreign to me — they are not owned by me and I can tell that it is the Devil, since their quality shows it', then the diagnosis of schizophrenia must be entertained. Alan should be asked to explain how he knows it is the Devil, and how anyone has the power to put thoughts into one's mind; in addition, he should be asked about what the experience of interference feels like, and whether the Devil causes the rituals as well as the thoughts.

Several points must be borne in mind in this assessment. Firstly, belief in the Devil as an actual entity is not, in itself, delusional in religious cultures. Alan has been brought up in a relatively strict Christian tradition — although not a fundamentalist one — which would make his belief in the Devil's existence compatible with his culture. Secondly, since obsessional ruminations and rituals can be seen as an attempt to 'parcel off' less controlled and less pleasant urges — of an aggressive or sexual kind — then it is understandable that those suffering from them explain them as having nothing to do with the 'real me'. Finally, if it is decided that Alan is indeed describing thought insertion and/or delusions of passivity, it is important to be sure that he has no other psychotic phenomena such as auditory hallucinations or a secondary delusional system.

13

Anxiety

Anxiety is one of the subjective emotions which corresponds to an increased level of psychological arousal. It is experienced normally and appropriately at times of stress when the resulting physiological and psychological changes are adaptive. However, there are times when the development and presence of anxiety is pathological, when it exists over and above the level which is normally considered appropriate to the situation. In these circumstances patients may present with psychological or somatic symptoms or a combination of the two, and the anxiety may be free-floating as in anxiety neurosis, or situation-specific as in phobic neurosis, or both; and may be discrete in itself or part of another psychiatric disorder.

ANXIETY STATES

Epidemiology

Anxiety states probably constitute the commonest form of psychiatric illness in highly developed countries, with a prevalence ranging from 2–5% of the general population of this country, to nearly 25% warranting professional help in the United States, where psychological illness is perhaps more acceptable. There is an equal sex incidence, with age of onset in the mid-twenties. There are both genetic and environmental factors in the aetiology.

Symptoms

As stated above, symptoms may be psychic (see Table 13.1) or somatic (see Table 13.2) or a mixture of the two. One common distressing psychic symptom of anxiety is *depersonalization* in which the person feels that she is no longer her

Table 13.1 Psychic symptoms of anxiety

The feeling of anxiety
Inability to relax
Initial insomnia
Inability to concentrate
Irritability
Fears of impending doom
Depersonalization

normal self. She may complain that she feels unreal, or is unable to feel anything or is floating out of her body looking down on herself from above. It is often accompanied by *derealization* in which the environmental surroundings are experienced as flat, dull and unreal.

Of the somatic symptoms, breathlessness is often described as an inability to get enough air into the body accompanied by a gasping or choking feeling. Objectively, the patient can be seen to be hyperventilating with irregular respiratory rhythm punctuated by sighs and pauses. Chest pain may be experienced as sharp, left inframammary pain or as a diffuse heavy sensation over the whole of the precordium, and may be associated with functional ECG changes — T-wave inversion and ST depression. Tension headaches

Table 13.2 Somatic symptoms of anxiety

Palpitations
Breathlessness
Chest pain
Headache
Paraesthesiae
Trembling
Fatigue
Sweating
Flushes
Dry mouth
Frequency of micturition

are usually felt as a tight band around the head and disturbance of consciousness, with lightheadedness, faintness and dizziness are frequent complaints, and some patients may also describe 'fits' (see Chapter 20). Motor disturbances may include tremor, restlessness, fidgeting or agitation; pain and paraesthesiae may occur.

Panic attacks occur when the patient experiences intense fear accompanied by high autonomic nervous system output, during which she may feel that she is going to die and may be compelled by an overwhelming desire to run away, or be rooted to the ground paralyzed by fear.

The somatic symptoms are themselves intensely anxiety-provoking so that by the time the patient presents a vicious circle has been set up and the anxiety state becomes self-perpetuating, with the initial precipitating cause, often a loss or threatened loss, or marital or occupational problem, long gone (see Figure 1).

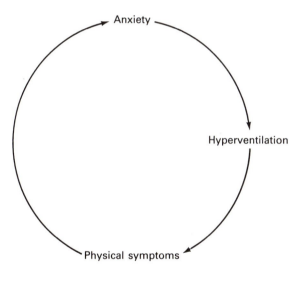

Figure 1

Physiology

There are both peripheral and central physiological components to anxiety. Peripherally the autonomic nervous system is activated with increased sympathetic activity leading to an increase in heart rate and blood pressure, a redis-

tribution of blood favouring the muscles, increased sweating and decreased salivation, and dilation of pupils and pilomotor erection. Muscle tension is increased, leading to pain and fatigue, and there is often an increased tremor. Respiration alters to produce hyperventilation with a rapid rate and irregular rhythm leading to a decrease in PCO_2. This causes a reduction in cerebral oxygenation both via cerebral vasoconstriction and the Bohr effect, leading to such neurological symptoms as lightheadedness, confusion, and occasionally, in susceptible patients, epileptic fits. Changes in calcium ionization cause neuromuscular irritability with, in extreme cases, tetany, and the increased respiratory use of thoracic musculature produces chest pain. Endocrine changes in anxiety include an increase in plasma cortisol and urinary steroid excretion, and a rise in adrenalin production. New experiences cause anxiety as a normal response but whereas normal people usually adapt or habituate to new stimuli and cease to show physiological responses, anxious patients fail to adapt and continue to react to repeated exposure to the stimulus.

Measurements

Various physiological parameters such as pulse rate, regional blood flow, salivation and sweating can be measured, and this is used both in research and clinical practice for diagnosis and treatment. However all that these measurements demonstrate is the level of arousal which ranges in any individual from sleep to excitement and does not indicate the specific emotion involved. Centrally the expression of anxiety is mediated by the limbic system and reticular formation. The latter is reflected by an increase in fast wave beta and the lack of slow alpha activity in the EEG.

Questionaires can be used to measure anxiety, ranging from a simple fear thermometer which is an analogue scale filled in by the patient, to more complicated questionaires such as the Taylor Manifest Anxiety Scale, the Hamilton Anxiety Rating Scale and the Zung Self-Assessment Rating Scale. Fear questionaires can be used in the evaluation of phobias, and in addition questionaires which assess behaviour and emotional response to target phobic situations are useful.

Differential diagnosis

The differential diagnosis is from both physical and psychiatric disorders. Physically thyrotoxicosis, phaeochromocytoma, carcinoid tumour and temporal lobe epilepsy have to be considered. In addition the group of symptoms with which the patient presents may suggest organic pathology, most commonly neurological (headache, light-headedness, 'fits') or cardiac (chest pain, breathlessness). Usually a full history will indicate the correct diagnosis since the development of anxiety symptoms is a pattern that should be immediately recognized, but in some circumstances investigations may be needed to rule out physical illness. The danger of over-investigation is that it may become increasingly difficult to convince the patient that he is suffering from a psychological illness. Where it is considered that the patient's symptoms may be due to hyperventilation it is often worth asking the patient to hyperventilate voluntarily to produce the same symptoms.

Psychiatrically, the most common diagnostic problem lies in deciding initially whether the patient's pathological anxiety is a sign of illness or is part of an underlying chronically anxious personality, or a combination of the two. Diagnosis of illness depends on being able to elicit the starting point of the disorder which must also represent a distinct and marked changes from *that patient's* normal state. If neither of the patient nor an informant can remember when he was any different then the anxiety is likely to be a manifestation of a personality disorder. Once one has established that the patient is suffering from a circumscribed illness it is necessary to decide whether the pathological anxiety is a discrete entity, namely an anxiety neurosis, or whether it is part of another psychiatric illness such as an acute confusional state or a schizophrenic illness. In these cases the diagnosis rests upon finding other associated signs suggestive of a wider disorder.

One of the commonest psychiatric disorders in which anxiety is a frequent symptom is depression, although it is not always possible to decide which is the primary mood disorder (see below).

Anxiety may lead to other difficulties with which the patient may present, such as alcoholism, where the alcohol is initially used as a tranquillizer; and sexual disorders, anxiety being one of the most common causes of performance failure. The anxious patient may become dependent on benzodiazepines prescribed for an apparently transient condition and may present for the first time to the psychiatrist when these drugs have been stopped.

Anxiety Psychosis

This is one of the cycloid psychoses (see Chapter 16).

Table 13.3 Classification of anxiety
Classification of pathological anxiety
Summarized from latest revisions of the International Classification of Disease (World Health Organisation, 1978) and Diagnostic and Statistical Manual of Mental Disorders (American Psychiatric Association, 1980)

ICD–9	DSM–III	Main diagnostic features
Acute stress reaction (308.0)	Post-traumatic stress disorder — acute (308.3)	Time-limited anxiety linked to marked stressful events
Adjustment reaction (309.2)	Post-traumatic stress disorder — chronic or delayed (309.81)	
Anxiety states (300.0)	Generalized anxiety disorder (300.02)	Non-situational anxiety
Phobic state (300.2)	Agoraphobia (300.22) Social phobia (300.23) Simple phobia (300.29) Agoraphobia with panic (300.21)	Situational anxiety
	Panic disorder (300.01)	Acute attacks of anxiety
Hypochondriasis (300.7)	Somatization disorder (300.81)	Somatic anxiety with fears of physical disease

Tyrer, P. (1984). Classification of anxiety. *British Journal of Psychiatry*, **144**, 78–83.

Table 13.4 Differences Between Anxiety Neurosis And Related Disorders In Which Anxiety Is A Prominent Symptom

Key features	Anxiety Neurosis	Other Disorders
Duration of symptoms	Long-term with tendency to relapse	Acute stress and adjustment reactions are short-term and relapse is rare
Relationship to external stress	Episodes of increased symptoms related to stressful precipitants, but no close temporal relationship	Clear-cut temporal relationship between major external stress and symptoms (Acute stress and Post-traumatic stress disorder)
Additional symptoms	Secondary depressive, phobic and hypochondriacal symptoms common at times of greater anxiety	Anxiety symptoms common in depressive, obsessional, phobic and hypochondriacal neuroses but not persistent
Somatic symptomatology	Includes all types and grades of symptoms, provided psychic anxiety is also present	Somatic symptoms primary and not associated with autonomic arousal (Somatization disorder, hypochondriacal neuroses)
Premorbid personality	Abnormal, with dependent and asthenic features	Personality normal or if abnormal does not show dependent and asthenic features

Adapted from Tyrer, P. (1984). Classification of anxiety. *British Journal of Psychiatry*, **144**, 78–83.

CLASSIFICATION OF ANXIETY (see Tables 13.3 and 13.4).

Pathological anxiety may occur not only on its own but also in association with other psychiatric disorders. When it occurs as a discrete entity the diagnosis is anxiety neurosis, but when it occurs in association with other psychiatric disorders the diagnosis depends on the entire psychopathology; for example in the presence of phobias the diagnosis is phobic neurosis. While this has long been the case when anxiety is part of a schizophrenic, organic or phobic illness, even presentations which have until quite recently been diagnosed as anxiety neurosis have been reclassified. Where the primary presenting symptoms are somatic and not associated either with psychic symptoms or autonomic arousal then the diagnosis is hypochondriasis (ICD–9) or somatization disorder (DSM–III). DSM–III has gone one stage further and divorced panic attacks from the rubric of anxiety neurosis, reclassifying them as panic disorder. The causes and duration of the disorder is important, as anxiety following stress is also separately diagnosed as acute stress reaction and adjustment reaction in the ICD–9, and as post-traumatic stress disorder, acute, or chronic or delayed, in DSM–III. Classification is particularly complicated where anxiety and depression coexist in the absence of biological or psychotic symptoms,

suggesting a depressive illness, when it is not always possible to decide on the primacy of either mood state and where common sense but not international classification systems would suggest a diagnosis of mixed anxiety and depressive neurosis or state. However in the present classificatory systems the term anxiety neurosis forms the base of a diagnostic hierarchy and has assumed the status of first-line diagnosis much in the same way as paranoid illness.

PHOBIAS

Definition

A phobia can be defined as the presence of situation-specific anxiety which is out of proportion to the stress involved in the situation in which it occurs, cannot be explained or reasoned away and is beyond voluntary control; i.e. it is irrational, situation-dependent, pathological anxiety. The behavioural concomitant is avoidance of the feared situation(s). Clinically phobias are of relevance when they impair substantially the patient's lifestyle.

Epidemiology

Specific fears are common and normal in chilhood. Phobic symptoms in adulthood may, as in the case

Table 13.5 Classification of phobias

Class I: Phobias of external stimuli	Class II: Phobias of internal stimuli
Agoraphobia	Illness phobias
Social phobias	Obsessional phobias —
Animal phobias	classified under obsessional-
Miscellaneous specific phobias	compulsive neuroses

Adapted from Marks, I. M., *Fears and Phobias.* William Heinemann Medical Books Ltd, London.

of phobic neuroses, be dicrete entities or part of another psychiatric illness such as an affective disorder, an obsessive compulsive neurosis or schizophrenia. Phobic neuroses can be classified on the basis of either external stimuli or internal stimuli, or according to the nature of the stimulus itself (see Table 13.5). Table 13.6 compares patients with phobic disorders with those with anxiety states and with normal people, on various epidemiological and psychophysiological parameters.

Agoraphobia

Agoraphobia is also known as the 'housebound housewife' syndrome and is the commonest phobic neurosis, accounting for more than half of those presented. The phobic situations include shops, public places and transport and the fear is usually one of losing control or fainting in an embarrassing situation or in a place from which security cannot be easily reached — a point of no return. The anxiety is less if the person goes out accompanied, even by an inanimate object such as a shopping basket on wheels, or if she is in control of the situation, as when driving a car. Because

of the need to remove herself quickly and unobstrusively from the feared situation, aisle seats are often chosen at cinemas and theatres. The anxiety may be sufficiently intense to produce panic attacks leading to a phobic avoidance of these situations. Eventually the person becomes housebound, although some patients are also afraid of being alone at home and panic attacks may occur there too. Associated symptoms are free-floating anxiety, depersonalization and derealization; sexual and marital problems; personality difficulties; depressed mood; obsessive compulsive phenomena alcohol abuse and occasionally specific phobias. Sexual problems may precede the agoraphobia and marital problems may be caused both by the restrictions imposed by the disorder and also by the changes in the relationship following successful resolution of the symptoms.

Agoraphobia has a prevalence in the general population of about 0.6% and is commoner in women. The typical age of onset is the twenties, and onset is rare before the age of puberty or after forty. It may occur suddenly or gradually, usually in an anxious, obsessional, shy, or dependent personality, often with a history of childhood neurotic traits including school refusal. It tends to fluctuate in severity, with about a third of patients returning to normal; the prognosis being better with less severe phobias and with patients younger than the mid-thirties. The differential diagnosis includes anxiety states, depression, social phobia and personality abnormality, but a detailed history and mental state examination will distinguish these.

Table 13.6 Comparsion Between Anxiety States, Phobias And Normal Responses

	Anxiety state	Agroraphobia	Social phobia	Animal phobia	Normals
Women as a percentage	50	75	60	95	50
Age onset	25	24	19	4	-
Age treatment	36	32	27	30	-
Overt anxiety (0–6 scale)	2.6	2.0	2.0	0.4	0
Galvanic skin response spontaneous fluctuations	36	32	33	12	6
Galvanic skin response habituation rate	29	32	33	12	6
Resting forearm blood flow	4.8	2.9	2.6	2.2	2.0
Eyeblink conditioned response acquisition	11	15	19	21	14

Adapted from Marks, I. M., *Fears and Phobias.* William Heinemann Medical Books Ltd, London.

Social Phobias

People with social phobias feel anxious in social situations such as parties, crowded places, cinemas, theatres, restaurants or anywhere where they have to eat in public. They are afraid of having to speak in public, of people in authority, of being watched at work and of being critized in social situations. A common fear is that they will make a fool of themselves either by blushing or by vomiting in public. These fears lead to avoidance of social situations with particularly severe repercussions on their work and home life. Associated symptoms include depression; anxiety unrelated to the feared situation including other phobias; sexual problems; abnormal premorbid personalities; and alcohol abuse to relieve the phobic anxiety and the apprehension at the prospect of future encounters which, as with the agoraphobic, is often severe. It is slightly more common in women than in men, with the onset often in the late teens, either suddenly after an embarrassing social situation, or gradually as an extension of a sensitive premorbid personality. The differential diagnosis is from agoraphobia, anxiety state, depression, personality abnormality, poor social skills with secondary anxiety, and schizophrenia; but as with agoraphobia careful history-taking and mental state evaluation leads to the correct diagnosis.

Animal Phobias

Fear of animals is common and indeed normal in childhood but continues into adulthood in some people, mainly women, as an isolated phobia. These women are usually free from other psychiatric symptoms although there may be sexual dysfunction; they may have nightmares about the feared object.

Other Specific Phobias

These include fear of heights, flying, urinating or defaecating in public places. A fear of vomiting or observing others vomiting also occurs. Space phobia is a fear of falling in a situation where there is no source of support. Claustrophobia is a fear of being enclosed or shut in in such places as lifts, and is often part of a wider agoraphobic syndrome.

Illness Phobia

Some patients have fears that they might have a serious illness such as cancer. This tends to merge with hypochondriacal disorders. There are, however, other people whose specific phobias tend to be of hospital and medical treatment. Strictly speaking this is not a fear of illness but of its potential consequences and is more correctly classified as a phobia of external stimuli.

Obsessional Phobias

These are not direct fears but of the consequences of certain actions and are classified under obsessive compulsive neuroses

CASE HISTORY

BRENDA WALKER

Mrs Brenda Walker, a 33-year-old woman married for the second time, was referred by her general practitioner with a six-month history of being anxious all the time coupled with episodes of breathlessness, dizziness, pins and needles in her hands, a fear that she was going to faint and on occasion a feeling of unreality. These attacks occurred both at home and at work and although her employers were very caring and had offered her the use of a darkened room if she got one of her attacks, for the last three months she had been unable to work and had been on sick leave. She had been prescribed tranquillizers but although they had helped initially, she had found them much less useful of late and had stopped them abruptly just under three weeks before the appointment with her general practitioner, after watching a television pogramme describing their dangers. This had produced a marked worsening in her condition and it was at this state that she was referred urgently for a specialist opinion. She was seen the same day.

On further questioning the following story emerged. Brenda had been married at twenty-two to Mike, a man fifteen years older than she was whom she subsequently found out was dealing with drugs and stolen merchandise. He drank heavily and frequently shouted at her but had never hit her. After they had been married for five years he was sent to prison, having been convicted of a murder committed during the course of a business venture which had gone wrong. Brenda was both relieved to see the back of him and worried as to how she would cope without him. She visited him regularly in prison for the first two years. After two years she met Andrew, a company director who appeared on the surface very different from her husband. After one year they decided to get married and Brenda filed successfully for divorce. She did not tell Mike about this in person but wrote him a letter explaining the circumstances. He wrote back saying that he understood, would not fight the divorce and wished her luck. She had not heard from him or about him since then.

After Mike had been in prison for six years Brenda read a book in which a convicted murderer escaped from prison and killed his wife and children; it was around this time that she began to get very anxious. At about this time also she had begun to doubt whether Andrew really cared for her and was frightened in case he left her. Furthermore her elder brother, whom she idolized, had fallen out with her father whom she visited regularly, and she was caught in the middle passing messages from one to the other.

When discussing her childhood and family life it emerged that Brenda's parents had been very overprotective towards her and Brends's mother had herself been very nervous and had suffered from agoraphobia. When she first went to her secondary school Brenda had developed tummy aches which kept her off school. On all occasions physical examination had been negative but her mother continued to worry about her physical state. After leaving school she went to college to learn shorthand and typing. She had been at her present job ever since leaving college. She continued to live at home until she married Mike and had never even been away on holiday before that without her parents. At the age of twenty-nine she was involved in a road accident in which she sustained a head injury and was unconscious for nearly an hour.

At interview she appeared very tense and fidgety. She was obviously overbreathing and at one time asked to leave the room because she thought she was going to faint. She admited to being anxious but denied feeling depressed. She said that she had difficulty getting off to sleep and would lie awake for hours worrying. On waking in the morning she would feel something terrible was going to happen but did not know what it was.

Her husband, Andrew, was seen on his own and said that from what he knew Brenda had always been a worrier but that in the last six months she had become much worse. She often telephoned him at work asking him to come home quickly, saying that she thought she was going to die. At times she had urged him to call the general practitioner or take her to the local casualty department. He agreed that there had been some improvement initially from the tranquillizers but this had been shortlived and since stopping the drugs she had been even worse than before she started them. He said that he felt she was having a nervous breakdown and it was putting a tremendous strain on the marriage. He had thought of leaving her but had not told her this.

When the couple were seen together it soon became apparent that Brenda leaned on Andrew for support but that at times he seemed distant towards her and at others quite angry with her. She acknowledged that she was asking a lot of him but said that he was all she had and that he had married her for better or worse.

Brenda's brother was also seen and confirmed Andrew's opinion that Brenda had always been a worrier. He said that even as a child she was frightened and insecure and always used to tag along with him. He talked about the argument with his father and how Brenda seemed to need to repair the gulf between the two of them.

Questions

What diagnoses might account for Brenda's symptoms over the last six months and their exacerbation in the last two weeks?
How do Brenda's background, personality and previous experiences relate to her present condition?
Brenda presents with psychic and somatic symp-

toms of anxiety. Her breathlessness is due to hyperventilation as witnessed on examination, and this is responsible for the other physical symptoms. Her feelings of unreality are due to depersonalization associated with heightened anxiety, and may also be linked with her hyperventilation. However, though her symptoms are due to anxiety the diagnosis of an anxiety state depends on the anxiety not being attributable to real danger. Although it is theoretically possible that Mike might escape from jail and assault her, this is too remote a possibility to pose sufficient threat to account for the overwhelming anxiety experienced by her. Morever this anxiety is also focused on her present marriage and on her general health, as witnessed by the frequent request to her husband to organize medical attention. Finally the presence of panic attacks would, according to DSM–III, suggest a diagnosis not of anxiety neurosis but of panic disorder.

The other two possibilities which should be thought of to explain some of her symptoms are temporal lobe epilepsy and a drug withdrawal state following cessation of her minor tranquillizers in the two to three weeks prior to referral. The possible diagnosis of temporal lobe epilepsy would be raised by the feelings of unreality and if confirmed on an EEG might be related to her previous head injury. The fact that these symptoms are produced on hyperventilation is compatible with this diagnosis, and hyperventilation is often used to highlight epileptic foci on the EEG. However, both these other diagnoses, namely temporal lobe epilepsy and drug withdrawal, would be in addition to the main diagnosis of anxiety neurosis or panic disorder.

Brenda's mother's anxious nature may have genetically led to her daughter's being predisposed to pathological anxiety. In addition it would have had an environmental impact in her childhood, of providing an abnormal model of adult behaviour. Her parents' overprotectiveness, suggesting that the world was a place to be frightened of, might well have led to her being insecure, as reported by her brother. There is indeed evidence of abnormal anxiety in childhood in the episodes of school refusal and later on in life in the presence of an anxious personality. Furthermore the pattern of her two marriages suggests that the relationships she formed were of a dependent rather than a mature nature. This is also supported by her behaviour in the current family argument, showing an inability to tolerate and disruption in her previously dependable family set-up, a disruption to which either inaction or taking sides would inevitably lead.

Thus one can say that her constitution, childhood experiences and personality would have led her to be vulnerable to the development of anxiety state at times of threatened loss. In this case the threat was to her present relationship and the family harmony. Finally her lifelong feelings of insecurity, and the belief instituted in her by her parents that the world was a frightening place might well have led her to over-react when reading the book concerning the possible threat that her first husband might pose.

14

Sadness (Depression of mood)

The feeling of sadness or depression is one of the common symptoms with which patients present to doctors. Sadness, misery and despair are normal responses to adversity, but doctors are particularly concerned with pathological forms of depression or 'depressive illness'. However, the symptom of 'feeling depressed' occurs in a variety of psychiatric disorders and physical conditions; the differential diagnosis and classification of depression is therefore problematical.

Faced with the symptom of sadness, the doctor may need to make a series of diagnostic decisions: *1* to clarify whether this complaint is part of a pathological state, *2* to determine whether the pathological state amounts to a depressive syndrome or another psychiatric or physical disorder, and *3* to attempt to define what type of depressive syndrome is present. At the same time a formulation of the aetiological factors is made and an hypothesis constructed upon which a rational treatment plan is based.

The distinction between normal and pathological depression (Table 14.1) is made on the basis of the severity and duration of change in mood, and of the degree of impairment of the person's usual ability to look after himself and to cope with his responsibilities. Sometimes the quality of the depressed mood is quite different from the individual's usual experience of unhappiness, and this distinct quality is an important feature of some

forms of pathological depression. The judgment should also take account of the present circumstances of the person and his current problems, as well as what is known of his previous personality and his way of coping with stress in the past; in other words it depends upon the extent to which the 'depression' is a change from the individual's expected pattern of response. In many cases it is obvious both to the person affected and to those around him whether or not the depression is a 'normal' reaction to a loss suffered. Diagnostic difficulties arise either when depression occurs with a long delay after an adverse event, or after prolonged exposure to stress, or when the 'normal' reaction continues longer than expected. The

Table 14.1 'Normal' depression *V* pathological depression

1 Severity, duration and quality of the change in mood; and ability to function

2 Extent of change from the individual's expected pattern of response

3 Associated features of the 'depressive syndrome'

Table 14.2 Bereavement

Uncomplicated	Complicated by major depression
Numbness, unreality and denial followed by:	Retardation
Depressed moods	Prolongation
Poor appetite	Severe functional impairment
Weight loss	Ideas of worthlessness
Insomnia	Suicidal ideas
Poor concentration	Delusions
Guilt related to events surrounding the death, or blame of others	Hallucinations — May be unrelated to the loss
Physical symptoms Hallucinations — related to the loss	

pattern of other symptoms and signs accompanying the depressed mood will also help to determine whether the depresion is pathological or not. However, the case of bereavement illustrates that a syndrome rersembling depressive illness can occur as a normal reaction (Table 14.2).

THE SYNDROME OF DEPRESSIVE ILLNESS

The clinical picture of depressive illness can be very varied. The variation is in part related to differences in severity, but it is also useful to recognise different patterns of the depressive syndrome as they may differ in their response to treatment, and in their prognosis.

The commonest characteristics of the depressive syndrome are shown in Table 14.3 which shows the inclusion criteria for a 'major depressive episode' according to DSM–III. The central feature is a low mood with lack of enjoyment and reduced interest. The patient experiences a loss of energy and feels unable to complete his usual activities. This leads to a feeling of inability to cope, and may be expressed as a sense of helplessness, dependence on others or failure. There is an impairment in performance. This will usually

Table 14.3 Major depression: diagnostic criteria (DSM — III)

A Dysphoric mood, or loss of interest or pleasure

plus

B *At least four of the following:*
 1 Agitation or retardation
 2 Loss of energy, fatigue
 3 Loss of interest or pleasure, or loss of libido
 4 Feelings of worthlessness, self-reproach or inappropriate guilt
 5 Morbid thoughts, suicidal ideation
 6 Poor concentration, indeciveness
 7 Poor appetite/weight loss or increased appetite/weight gain
 8 Insomnia or hypersomnia

plus

C Duration: at least two weeks

affect appearance, giving an impression of self-neglect or poor grooming and dress. The facial expression is characterized by down-turned edges of the mouth and a furrowing between the eyebrows, associated with hunched shoulders and a slumped posture. This is partly under voluntary control and some patients are able to conceal their depressed feelings in their outward appearance.

There is a loss of interest or pleasure in things that he would normally enjoy. The sex drive is also reduced; in men this loss of libido leads to a diminution in sexual activity, whereas in women sexual activity may continue without enjoyment.

Psychomotor *retardation* involves a slowness of movement and speech. Gestures are weak or reduced, as are spontaneous movements such as blinking. There is a characteristic delay in replying to questions; this may last even for minutes before the patient replies and it is therefore liable to be overlooked if the assessment is hurried.

Agitation is a state of restlessness. The patient feels unable to relax and is seen to have repetitive movements, such as wringing hands, pulling fingers or hair, moving legs, inability to sit still, and leaving the chair or the room. Retardation and agitation may co-exist in the patient at the same time.

Thought content may be overwhelmingly depressive and the patient will view the past with a disproportionate sense of failure, self-reproach or guilt. In mild degrees this is shown as self-blame for letting the family down by being ill. In moderate cases the patient dwells on and magnifies events from the past for which he feels to blame (overvalued ideas of blame), whilst in severe cases the guilt reaches delusional proportions and the content may be bizarre. Occasionally it is difficult to distinguish between overvalued ideas and delusions of guilt. Thoughts about the present are dominated by loss of self-confidence and lowering of self-esteem, and by thoughts of failure or worthlessness. The patient may say that he does not deserve to be helped. The future is viewed with a sense of hopelessness. In mild cases the future can be contemplated, but only with a sense of inevitable failure. In moderate cases the future looks 'bleak' or 'black' while in severe depression the patient sees 'no future', or a future with well-deserved punishment or death. In this context it is important to enquire whether life seems worth living, or whether death would be welcomed, and to explore for thoughts or plans of self-harm. The further assessment of suicidal ideation and risk is considered elsewhere.

Depression is often accompanied by difficulty in concentration. The patient is most aware of this and may complain of poor concentration, such as inability to read his usual newspaper, or to watch a television programme; some patients express this as losing their memory, but formal testing shows that the forgetfulness is due mainly to poor registration of new information rather than to a defect in retention or recall. This inability to concentrate contributes to indecisivenes which is particularly liable to occur in obsessional personalities during depression.

Changes in somatic functions, including appetite and sleep, are frequent and of diagnostic importance. The change in appetite is usually in the direction of anorexia and is accompanied by weight loss and in severe cases by dehydration; a few patients experience increased appetite and gain weight. Likewise most patients complain of insomnia but a few sleep excessively; in both cases they tend to feel unrefreshed by sleep. In some cases, constipation is a problem.

In addition to the symptoms described so far, constituting the core of the depressive syndrome, depressive illness may be accompanied by other symptoms which are less specific and which occur more often in conditions other than depressive illness.

Phobic, obsessional and hysterical symptoms

Phobias and obsessions may develop during a depressive illness, either as an exacerbation of a pre-existing phobic or obsessional neurosis, or in the setting of an anxious or obsessional personality. There is an association between agoraphobia and depression, and social withdrawal and social phobias may also deteriorate. Patients with obsessional personalities are particularly predisposed to develop depression. Hysterical symptoms, in the form of hysterical conversion or dissociative phenomena, are often a response to underlying depressive illness. Depersonalization and fugue states are examples of symptoms which can develop in this way. The term depersonalization is used to describe both the absence of normal feelings in depression and the experience of being changed or even externalized from oneself, like an observer. Such phobic, obsessional and hysterical symptoms can be formulated as defence mechanisms that reduce depressive or anxious feelings.

Hallucinations and delusions

Severe depressive illness may be accompanied by delusions or hallucinations, which are characteristic in their content. Depressive delusions are concerned with ideas of personal inadequacy, guilt, hopelessness, or hypochondriasis. In some patients the delusions imply a denial of the existence either of a part of themselves, or of others, or of the world around them; these are called nihilistic delusions (Cotard's syndrome). Persecutory delusions may occur. These can arise either as an extension of ideas of guilt, such that punishment is expected; or alternatively, a pre-existing paranoid trait in the personality may provide the basis for delusional ideas to develop during depression. *Ideas of reference* consist of thoughts that incidental things that are heard or seen are especially directed at the patient. They occur mostly in those with 'sensitive' personalities, because of their tendency to brood, and their difficulty in externalizing feelings; such people are often both insecure and ambitious. During depression 'sensitive' persons are prone to develop more firmly held ideas of reference, or delusions of reference.

Auditory hallucinations may occur in severe depressive illness, taking the form of voices addressing the patient (in the second person) with a monotonous depressive content concerning his worthlessness, or his death. Some patients hear voices urging them to harm themselves. Sometimes patients recognize that these experiences are from their own imagination when they may be referred to as pseudo-hallucinations.

SUBTYPES OF MAJOR DEPRESSIVE DISORDER

It is sometimes possible to identify a particular type of depressive illness on the basis of the presenting symptoms and from the personal and family history. The subtypes of depressive illness are shown in Table 14.4. These syndromes are not all mutually exclusive.

Table 14.4 Subtypes of major depressive disorder

Melancholia (endogenous depression)

Bipolar depression

Recurrent unipolar depression

Retarded depression

Agitated depression

Depression with psychotic symptoms

Depression with reversed functional shift

Table 14.5 Melancholia: diagnostic criteria DSM — III

1 Loss of pleasure in all or almost all activities (anhedonia)

plus

2 Lack of reactivity to usually pleasurable stimuli (doesn't feel much better even temporarily when something good happens)

plus

3 At least three of the following:

  a Distinct quality of depressive mood i.e. the depressed mood is perceived as distinctly different from the kind of feeling experienced following the death of a loved one

  b The depression is regularly worse in the morning (diurnal variation)

  c Early morning awakening (at least two hours before the usual time of awakening)

  d Psychomotor retardation or agitation

  e Significant anorexia or weight loss

  f Excessive or inappropriate guilt

Melancholia

The term melancholia is used in DSM–III synonymously with the term 'endogenous depression'. In the past the term psychotic depression was used with the same meaning. Recognition of the syndrome depends mainly on the symptoms of physiological disturbance or 'functional shifts' as shown in Table 14.5. The diagnosis of this pattern of melancholic depression is often supported by evidence from the family and personal history. There may be a family history of major affective disorder, or a past history of an episode of major depression with full recovery and a relatively normal personality with few neurotic traits during the interval. Also this type of depressive episode may develop suddenly or without obvious precipitating factors, although in a majority of such episodes a precipitant is reported.

Bipolar depression

Patients with a major depressive episode who have also experienced an episode of mania are classified as bipolar (manic-depressive) disorder depressed. A distinction is made between patients who have a history of an episode meeting the full diagnostic criteria for mania (bipolar 1) and those who have experienced an episode of pathologically elevated mood (often occurring during the recovery from depression with treatment) with some features of mania, but not of sufficient duration or severity to meet the full diagnostic criteria. The latter has been called bipolar II, or atypical bipolar disorder (DSM–III). The clinical presentation of bipolar depression is similar in symptom-profile to that of unipolar depression, although there is a tendency for less anxiety, agitation and somatic complaints in the bipolar group.

Unipolar depression

The term unipolar depression is generally reserved for patients who have recurrent episodes of major depression, usually with melancholic features, and without mania. These patients may be subdivided into retarded or agitated depressives, if the psychomotor changes are sufficiently marked. A severely retarded depression, if untreated, may develop into a depressive stupor. In some cases agitation dominates the clinical picture; depression of mood may be less prominent than the sense of unease, and it is often accompanied by hypochondriacal ideas or delusions, and a monotonous search for reassurance, which has been called importuning.

In some patients symptoms of both depression and mania coexist and the diagnostic category used in these cases is mixed affective state (see Chapter 16).

Depression with psychotic features

Although the presence of depressive delusions or auditory hallucinations justifies the label psychotic depression, the latter term has also been used in cases where the depressive thought content is not of delusional intensity but does reveal an impaired sense of reality and loss of insight. Certain psychotic features are regarded as consistent with depression of mood (mood-congruent) as revealed by the content of the delusions or hallucinations. The mood-congruent depressive themes include ideas of personal inadequacy, guilt, disease, death, nihilism, or deserved punishment. The auditory hallucinations are typically brief, and words are experienced in the second person, addressing the patient. If the psychotic symptoms have a content that does not involve these depressive themes, they are regarded as 'mood-incongruent'. If the form of the psychotic features corresponds to one of the 'first-rank symptoms' of Schneider they are best regarded as mood-incongruent, irrespective of their content. This is because the coexistence of depressive symptoms with schizophrenia is far commoner than the occurrence of such schizophrenic symptoms in depressive illness.

In some patients it is not possible either to differentiate with any degree of certainty between affective disorder and schizophrenia or to place them in any other diagnostic category; they are diagnosed as suffering from schizoaffective disorder.

Depression with reversed functional shift

In some patients the episode of depressive illness is accompanied by changes in biological functions, the opposite of those associated with melancholia. Thus there may be an increase in appetite and weight gain, together with exessive sleeping and tiredness rather than insomnia. The syndrome may occur as part of a bipolar disorder. In 'seasonal affective disorder', depression of this type occurs in the dark winter months and is succeeded by a mild manic state when the weather is brighter in the summer.

DIFFERENTIAL DIAGNOSIS OF MAJOR DEPRESSIVE DISORDER

Difficulties in diagnosis arise either when non-specific symptoms dominate the clinical presentation so that the depressive syndrome is evident only when specific enquiries are made (masked depression), or when the depression of mood is prominent but other symptoms of the depressive syndrome are not.

Masked depression

Sometimes difficulty arises because the patient presents with physical symptoms, or complains of difficulties in life, and does not mention a depressed mood until this is asked about. He may not equate the abnormal feelings of depressive illness with sadness. In other cases another symptom that may or may not be part of the depressive syndrome dominates and the change in mood is less prominent.

Patients with an obsessional personality type tend to control or suppress their feelings, making the recognition of a lowered mood difficult. Other people can hide their depression behind a cheeful facade (smiling depression). These patients may, however, come to tears when listened to in a sympathetic manner. Schizoid personalilteies are prone to depressive depersonalization with accompanying anxiety about their extinction or about madness. Terms other than sadness or depression may be used by the patient to describe his altered mood. Anxiety, irritability, pessimism, apathy, or feelings or emptiness may occur. Sometimes they express a loss of feeling and a sense of deadness or remoteness; this is one form of depersonalization. Paranoid personalities are likely to project some of their feelings and thoughts, and to express grievances. Phobic or obsessional symptoms may develop in association with depression and may be the presenting complaint.

Psychomotor retardation or agitation may so impair concentration that the patient is forgetful. His own awareness of this is usually greater than the deficit that is apparent on clinical examination, but sometimes the condition may be difficult to distinguish from organic intellectual deterioration; this is called *pseudodementia*. The examination of higher cerebral functions will not reveal dysphasia, agnosia, or dyspraxia as in true dementia. Moreover the demented patient is less likely to complain of memory failure, owing to lack of insight.

It may be behaviour associated with depression which bring the patient to medical attention. For instance, self-neglect or inability to cope in the home or at work; or antisocial behaviour, such as shoplifting; or rarely sexual indiscretion, or aggressive behaviour, or alcohol or stimulant drug abuse.

Somatic complaints (See Chapter 21)

Depressed patients often complain about physical symptoms. These complaints arise in various ways. The patients may be preoccupied with one of the somatic features of depression, such as anorexia, weight loss, constipation, insomnia, loss of libido, loss of energy, or somatic anxiety. The patient may begin to worry that he has a physical disease, such as cancer of the bowel or brain, or venereal disease. Alternatively he may dwell gloomily on some normal feature of his body that he has not previously noticed or worried about. Muscular tension accompanying depression or anxiety can lead to pain, especially frontal or occipital headache or facial pain, and to a sensation of tightness of chest which may be associated with sighing, or hyperventilation, and complaints of breathlessness. Any previous physical illness may also become a focus for a depressive preoccupation. These somatic preoccupations may take the form of obessional ruminations, phobic

anxiety or overvalued ideas, or hypochondriacal delusions.

LESS SEVERE OR PERVASIVE DEPRESSIVE SYNDROMES (Table 14.6)

Less severe or pervasive depressive syndromes may represent either a residual phase of a major depressive episode, or a mild depressive mood swing in a person prone to subclinical depressive and/or manic episodes — cyclothymia. Alternatively it may represent a state of emotional distress resembling major depression, but not as severe. This is called '*dysthymic disorder*', a term which is used in DSM–III as an alternative to 'depressive neurosis', or neurotic depression in ICD-9 (Table 14.7). The requirement for a duration of two years may be too stringent and it is perhaps more appropriate to distinguish between brief and chronic states of dysthymia (or morbid distress).

The difficulty in determining whether a group of depressive symptoms is pathological or is a normal reaction to loss has already been discussed in the context of bereavement. When the 'loss' is less severe than, for instance, the death of someone close, there will normally be a transient 'adjustment reaction', which will normally be accompanied by a period of impairment in function and depression of mood, with or without tearfulness and pessimistic thoughts but not other symptoms. This would be classified as an 'adjustment disorder with depressed mood'.

Table 14.6 Less severe or pervasive depressive syndromes

1 Cyclothymia
2 Dysthymic disorder
3 Bereavement
4 Adjustment disorder with depressed mood
5 Symptomatic depression
6 Depression in another psychiatric disorder

DEPRESSIVE COGNITION

In some patients depression of mood may be caused or maintained by certain errors of thinking, which distort the person's perception of

Table 14.7 Dysthymic disorder (depressive neurosis): diagnostic criteria

1 Duration: At least 2 years, but not severe enough for major depression

plus

2 Intervals free of depression not more than a few months

plus

3 Depressed mood or loss of interest

plus

4 At least three of the following:
   a Insomnia or hypersomnia
   b Low energy or tiredness
   c Low self-esteem
   d Reduced capacity to work
   e Poor concentration
   f Social withdrawal
   g Loss of interest
   h Irritability
   i Inability to respond with pleasure
   j Less talkative
   k Pessimism
   l Tearfulness
   m Morbid thoughts

reality. Four basic types of errors may be identified and be a focus for treatment with cognitive thereapy. These are:

1 Arbitrary inference: conclusions are drawn on the basis of subjective impressions alone.
2 Selective abstraction: particular details of a complex situation are focused on while others are ignored.
3 Overgeneralization: conclusions about personal ability or worth are drawn on the basis of a single incident.
4 Minimization and magnification: gross inaccuracies are made in judging the significance of events, so that actual performance is underestimated, or problems are overestimated.

Evidence of these depressive cognitions can be obtained by asking the patient to verbalize the 'automatic thought' that goes rapidly through his mind shortly before he reacts to internal or external events by feeling depressed.

CULTURAL FACTORS

Culture may influence the way in which depressive disorders present, and may also play a pathogenic or a protective role in the causation of depression. Some African and Asian cultures express depression mainly through somatic complaints, or ideas of a paranoid kind rather than guilt. Language difficulties may alter the meaning of words describing states of feelings. There may be differences in body image and symbolism; for instance loss of libido may be equated with weakness of the back. Heartache may refer to loss of feelings for close relations. In countries where medicine is predominantly techincal, the performance of a series of investigations with negative results may reinforce the patient's anxiety that a serious physical disease is present.

Guilt feelings seem to be especially common in depression in Judaeo-Christian cultures. In other cultures there is a greater tendency to projection either on to the family group or on to God; in the latter case the concept of divine retribution does imply some idea of wrongdoing. Some religions regard suicide as a major sin and this may affect the incidence of actual suicide.

The role of the individual in the family group varies between cultures, and this may affect the role of life-events in producing depression. Moreover rapid changes in cultural patterns of support may render the individual more vulnerable to depression at times of stress, through the absence of the expected empathy from relatives. The roles of men and women differ according to culture and are changing. In some cultures the role of women is still considered to be solely marriage and motherhood, and failure in this or death of a husband may have a quite different significance from that in other cultures, where the idea of failure, worthlessness or helplessness would not be encouraged. Male depressives are more likely than females to resist the impulse to cry.

AGE

Although depression of mood is common in adolescence, the syndrome of major depression is unusual then. When it does occur it may represent the onset of a recurrent bipolar or unipolar affective disorder. However, when depression with psychotic features occurs in late adolescence or early adult life without a family history of affective disorder, it may presage the onset of a schizophrenic illness.

The profile of the depressive syndrome differs somewhat according to age. Younger patients are more likely to experience hypersomnia than insomnia, and to appear irritable, disagreeable and intolerant.

The term involutional melancholia was formerly used to describe agitated depression developing for the first time after the age of about 50 (or 60 in men) in persons with previously rigid, obsessional personality traits. The usefulness of this separate category is now doubted, although elderly depressed patients tend to present with more agitation, hypochondriasis and initial insomnia than younger depressives. In patients whose depressive illness occurs for the first time in late adulthood, there is less likely to be a positive family history of affective illness and there may be indications of minor degrees of organic cerebral pathology predisposing to depression, due either to the ageing process or to cerebral vascular disease.

THE HISTORY

In assessing depressive symptoms it is important to establish whether any recent major 'life-events' have occurred; particularly adverse events, including 'losses'. Such losses may be real, threatened or imagined, and may involve loss of a relationship through bereavement or separation, a change of occupation or environment, financial loss, or loss of some role or ideal. As well as recent events, early losses, particularly of parents in childhood, may be relevant in determining the individual's response to loss in adulthood.

A family history of psychiatric disorder, especially of affective illness or suicide, may be relevant and indicate a genetic contribution to the aetiology. Bipolar depression has a strong genetic basis, but the relatives of bipolar patients show also a high rate of unipolar depression. Bipolar II disorder appears to breed true in some families,

rather than being solely a milder manifestation of bipolar I disorder. Other forms of depression with less marked physiological disturbances appear to be linked with a family history of alcoholism and antisocial behaviour disorder.

It is important to determine the extent of drug and alcohol consumption and to examine for physical illness. The previous personality should be assessed, especially with regard to mood traits suggestive of cyclothymia, previous responses to adversity, and traits that may predispose to depression, such as obsessional traits or dissociative tendencies. It is also important to assess the support currently available. Housebound individuals with several young children and without a close confiding relationship are particularly vulnerable to depressive states (mostly dysthymic disorders) and these may be exacerbated by a new 'loss'.

Any evidence of another, coexisting, mental disorder such as schizophrenia, personality disorder, anorexia nervosa or alcoholism should be elicited, as should evidence of sexual deviation, or gambling. If there is a recent history of antisocial behaviour, it may be necessary to assess the extent to which the onset of depressive symptoms antedated the incident or offence.

In depression in the year following childbirth the history should include questions about complications of pregnancy and delivery and the mother's attitude to childbirth, as these may in some cases be more relevant to the depressive symptoms than are the hormonal changes which are thought to produce the early *maternity blues* and in some cases to precipitate the more severe or psychotic forms of puerperal mental disorder.

It must be remembered that no assssessment of a depressed patient is complete without a thorough understanding of the extent of the risk of suicide.

SYMPTOMATIC DEPRESSION

A depressive state may develop following a clear physical disturbance by drugs (or drug withdrawal) or by disease. The drugs most likely to do this are those which interact with the biogenic amine neurotransmitters (noradrenaline, dopamine, 5-HT, or ACh) or with the enzyme co-factors (especially B vitamins and folic acid) involved in their synthesis. Some drugs may cause depression in patients with no evidence of a predisposition to affective disorders in the family history or past psychiatric history. However, a predisposition to depression does seem to render an individual more liable to develop a major depressive syndrome when certain drugs are taken. The drugs most commonly incriminated are shown in Table 14.8. Other commonly prescribed drugs, such as anti-inflammatory analgesics and diuretic drugs, may cause a lowering of spirits in some individuals.

Physical disease may be followed by depression and several mechanisms may be involved (Table 14.9). Those diseases making the most psychological impact are diseases affecting such vital organs as the heart, or such symbolically important organs as the uterus and breasts, or diseases such as cancer. However. the diseases or organs linked directly with the central nervous system are more likely to cause depression by organic mechanisms. When a full depressive syndrome occurs in response to disease in an individual with no family or past history of depressive illness, the condition is called 'organic depressive disorder' or 'symptomatic depression'.

The physical conditions most likely to be accompanied by depression are shown in Table 14.10. The nature of the depressive state accompanying these conditions varies.

Drugs and endocrine or metabolic disorders are more likely to precipitate a full depressive syndrome in predisposed individuals; in persons

Table 14.9 Mechanisms by which physical disease may cause depression

1 Psychological reaction to loss of health, function or independence
2 Response to chronic pain
3 Disease impairs coping mechanisms
4 Disease produces symptoms that are part of depressive syndrome
5 Disease causes full major depressive syndrome

Table 14.8 Drugs and Depression

Cardiovascular drugs	Others
reserpine	disulfiram
Alpha-methyldopa	barbiturates
beta blockers (propranolol, metoprolol)	indomethacin
	anticholinesterases

Steroids
corticosteroids
oral contraceptives

Withdrawal of stimulants and appetite suppressants
amphetamines
fenfluramine
diethylpropion
phenmetrazine

Neurological drugs
L-dopa
bromocriptine
baclofen
tetrabenazine
phenytoin

Antimicrobials
co-trimoxazole
isoniazid
cycloserine

Table 14.10 Symptomatic depression

Neurological	Endocrine
cerebral arteriosclerosis	myxoedema
arteriosclerotic dementia	thyrotoxicosis
Alzheimer's dementia	Cushing's syndrome
head injury	Addison's disease
stroke	hypoparathyroidism
subdural haematoma	pseudo-hypoparathyroidism
subarachnoid haemorrhage	
cerebral tumour	
Parkinson's disease	*Metabolic*
multiple sclerosis	
temporal lobe epilepsy	acute intermittent porphyria
narcolepsy	folate deficiency
Kleine-Levin syndrome	B12 deficiency
	hypercalcaemia
Infectious	
	Carcinoma
Viral	
influenza	pancreas
hepatitis	medullary carcinoma of
infective mononucleosis	thyroid
encephalitis	
Bacterial	*Auto immune*
neurosyphilis	disseminated lupus
toxoplasmosis	erythematosus
brucellosis	temporal arteritis
Genetic	
Huntington's chorea	
Kleinfelter's syndrome	

who are not predisposed, the disease or drug may cause a lowering of mood together with other depressive symptoms (e.g. anorexia, weight loss, tiredness, apathy, insomnia, poor concentration) but not an extensive depressive syndrome. In patients with structural brain damage, sites of cerebral impairment are probably more important than predisposition.

The clue to the underlying organic nature of the depression may be that there are symptoms likely to be organic in origin such as occasional disorientation or memory impairment, or cognitive impairments such as dysphasia, agnosia or dyspraxia. Physical examination may reveal neurological abnormalities or other signs of physical disease.

A full physical examination is therefore indicated in any depressed patient whose condition does not appear fully explicable in psychological terms. Laboratory tests should include a full blood count, ESR, urea and electrolytes, liver function test, fasting calcium, folate, B12 and cortisol levels, antinuclear factor and serology for syphilis. X-rays of the chest and skull may also be required as may an EEG or CAT scan. A lumbar puncture may be necessary for the diagnosis of neurosyphilis. Urine examination and testing for proteins, ketones and sugar is indicated. Special testing for virology and porphyria may be indicated, as may temporal artery biopsy.

DEPRESSION WITH ANOTHER PSYCHIATRIC DISORDER

The conditions listed in Table 14.11 are commonly accompanied by depressed mood, and may even predispose to the development of a major depressive episode.

Depressive symptoms may presage the onset of *schizophrenia*, or depression may become manifest

Table 14.11 Psychiatric disorders with a secondary depression

1 Schizophrenia
2 Dementia
3 Alcoholism
4 Personality disorder: histrionic type 　　　　　　　　　　　　 borderline type

after recovery from an acute schizophrenic episode (post-psychotic depression). This may occur either as a new development, or as an emergence of depression from a mixed clinical picture when schizophrenic symptoms have subsided ('revealed depression'). Similarly a patient with a history of acute schizophrenic breakdown may present with acute depressive symptoms in the course of long-term treatment with antipsychotic medication. A state resembling retarded depression can develop in association with drug-induced Parkinsonism when the patient feels dysphoric and immobile. This is particularly liable to happen in the first week after injections of depot anti-psychotic medication ('akinetic depression').

Emotional lability, or sudden crying as part of a catastrophic reaction may occur in *dementia* and suggest frontal lobe brain damage. Depression may occur in the early stage of dementia before the cognitive impairment becomes obvious, although the true diagnosis may only be made with hindsight.

Alcohol abuse or dependence may occur secondarily to depression and this may be especially relevant in middle-aged females with alcoholism. Alternatively, alcoholism may predispose to depression through the effects of the drug, and may also be genetically associated with an increased risk of depression. Alcholism is an important risk factor for suicidal acts in depression.

Personality disorders may predispose to depressive illness, but difficulties in differential diagnosis arise when depressive mood swings are a prominent feature of the person's reaction to stress. Thus patients with histrionic personalities may given exaggerated displays of emotion in reaction to events, and those with borderline personalities show marked changes of mood of brief duration accompanying intense and unstable relationships. In both cases the abnormalities of mood are characteristic of their long-term functioning and are not limited to episodes of illness.

LABORATORY TESTS IN DEPRESSIVE ILLNESS

There is hope that advances in molecular biology may soon lead to genetic probes that may identify

Table 14.12 Biological markers of depressive illness

Trait markers

1 Reduced CSF level of 5HT metabolite 5HIAA

2 Blunting of growth hormone response noradrenaline alpha-2 agonist drug clonidine

3 Increased sensitivity to the suppressant effect of bright light upon nocturnal melatonin secretion

4 Increased sensitivity to the induction of REM sleep by cholinergic agonist drug arecoline

State markers

1 Increased circulating cortisol levels throughout 24 hours

2 Resistance of circulating cortisol level to suppression by dexamethasone (dexamethasone suppression test)

3 Blunting of thyrotrophin (TSH) response to thyrotrophin-releasing hormone (TRH)

4 Reduced melatonin levels in blood

the susceptibility to affective disorder, and thereby assist in diagnosis. At present there are only a few accepted biological markers of either the predisposition (trait-markers) or the state of depressive illness (state-markers) (see Table 14.12). The value of these markers will depend upon their sensitivity (the proportion of cases that show the abnormality) and their specificity for the disorder in question, as compared with other disorders or normal subjects. None of these can at present be recommended for routine use in diagnosis, although they are of great research interest.

CASE HISTORY

JOHN EVANS

Mr John Evans, a 63-year-old married former coalminer, was referred for a psychiatric opinion by his general practitioner following his wife's complaints that all he did all day was sit at home in his chair looking miserable. Mr Evans had first noticed a change in his mood shortly after a heart attack one year previously, which had resulted in his premature retirement. At about the same time his elder brother, who had a history of angina pectoris, had died suddenly whilst mowing the lawn. He had been very close to this brother, whom he had regarded as his best friend, and had been devastated by his death.

He had become depressed and anxious, and worried that he too might soon be dead. He was preoccupied with his health and complained frequently of chest pain and breathlessness, which were not characteristic of myocardial ischaemia. He had difficulty sleeping, his nights were disturbed and he woke an hour and a half earlier than normal, after which he lay in bed brooding and unable to return to sleep. He had frequent nightmares about his time as a prisoner-of-war in Burma. He had thought a lot about the friends he had lost, as well as his father who had died when he was five, his brother who had been killed during the war, and a daughter who had died from meningitis at the age of two. When he talked about these losses, tears came into his eyes. He admitted that he had never before been able to cry over them.

His wife said he had lost weight and he agreed that he was no longer interested in food. Prior to this he and his wife had had an active and enjoyable sex-life but he could no longer be bothered with this area of his life. He had always enjoyed a pint of beer and a game of dominoes in the pub with his friends, but he had hardly been out with them at all in the last six months. Previously a keen and regular churchgoer, he now spent Sunday mornings in his chair at home, feeling there was little point in praying. He had no energy, interest, or ability to concentrate, even on television programmes, and just sat in his chair for long periods looking vacant. His wife complained that he often did not answer questions, particularly over the last month, and she had noticed that he appeared very slow in his actions. Mr Evans agreed with this and added that his thinking had slowed up and his memory was awful.

His mental state revealed a retarded but reasonably groomed man, although it later transpired that this was a result of his wife's caring and if left to his own devices he would not have shaved or washed. He looked much older that his years and had obviously lost weight. There was no spontaneous speech and he took a long time to answer questions. He admitted to being depressed and said that he felt that there was no future; he was useless and a burden to his wife and children and they'd be better off if he were dead. On further questioning he said that he had thought on a number of occasions in the last few days of ending it all but could not summon up the energy to do so. He cried when talking about his losses and said that nowadays he often dwelt on sad events in the past. He denied any delusions of guilt or persecution and there was no evidence of auditory hallucinations. He was well orientated, and when made to concentrate, showed no evidence of cognitive impairment.

He had been born in Wales, the son of a coalminer who committed suicide, after a third bout of depression, when the patient was five. His paternal grandfather had also suffered with depression. His mother remarried when he was eight and he got on well with his stepfather. His early childhood was uneventful and he did well at school. After leaving school he followed the family tradition and became a coalminer, a job he enjoyed. He married a local girl at the age of twenty-three and it appeared to have been a happy marriage. During the war he served in the Far East and spent three years in a Japanese P.O.W. camp. On his return he did not talk about his experience but resumed his prewar life-style. His premorbid personality was described as anxious and obsessional and he always bottled up his feelings. There was no evidence of alcohol abuse. Ten years ago he had become depressed following a threat of redundancy and this had responded to antidepressants.

Questions

What is the diagnosis?
What are the aetiological factors?

The signs and symptoms of depressed and hopeless mood with ideas of uselessness, grief and suicide; psychomotor retardation; tearfulness; loss of interests, appetite, weight and libido; early morning waking and nightmares; anergia; poor concentration; lack of personal hygiene; social withdrawal; these are classical symptoms of a major depressive illness. This is supported by the family history of depression and his own previous episode.

In a man with these symptoms, family and past history, there is no differential diagnosis. However, one could argue that this may initially have started as a pathological grief reaction, or anxiety, secondary to the deterioration in his physical health.

The most important aetiological factors are his genetic predisposition to depression and his history of losses. The death of his father at the age of five may have increased his vulnerability to the effect of losses. Further important bereavements occurred during a time of particular stress (the War), when he was unable to grieve. His personality would, even in favourable circumstances, have made normal grieving and coping with loss difficult.

His previous episode of depression followed a threatened loss and this illness follows closely upon the death of his brother, and his loss of health and usefulness as a working man. He also has cause to be anxious that he may suffer sudden death as did his brother. His chest pain and breathlessness may not only be a manifestation of this anxiety but also part of the grieving process for his brother, with whom he identifies.

15

Suicide, parasuicide and self-mutilation

DEFINITIONS

Suicide is the act of deliberately taking one's own life. parasuicide is deliberate self-injury whether or not the motive is suicide and is therefore a better term than attempted suicide. There is a third circumscribed group of repetitive self-mutilators (see below).

EPIDEMIOLOGY

Suicide has both legal and religious connotations. Historically, as suicide was a sin, a person who had died by this means was not allowed to be buried amongst his peers. Attempted suicide used to be considered a crime but this is no longer the case, although assisting a suicide attempt remains illegal. Nevertheless, the recent increase in interest in euthanasia for the incurably ill has led to debate concerning the morality of this law.

Estimates of the suicide rate from coroners' inquests are probably low since this verdict is only reached when the evidence for suicide is beyond doubt. The suicide rate has fallen in England and Wales in the last twenty years from about fifteen to eight per 100,000. There is evidence that this has now levelled off and is now increasing. This fall is most pronounced in elderly males while in elderly females the reverse is true. Reasons for this decrease may include the change from coal gas to non-toxic North Sea gas, the use of nonlethal minor tranquillizers in place of the more dangerous barbiturates and the development of psychiatric services and methods of treatment.

In contrast, the rate of parasuicide has risen dramatically over the same period of time, though there are signs that this too is levelling off. It has reached such epidemic proportions that it now represents the commonest reason for an emergency medical admission to the general hospital in young adults. Rates vary greatly with age and sex and many cases go undetected or unreported so that it is difficult to give an overall rate but it is likely to be in the hundreds per 100,000.

PROFILES

The profiles of suicide and parasuicide patients are very different, as shown in Table 15.1. The patient who successfully commits suicide is statistically more likely to be a middle-aged to elderly man of high social class, single, divorced or widowed, often recently bereaved, socially isolated, unemployed or retired, chronically physically ill and suffering from a psychiatric illness, usually depression or alcoholism. In contrast a patient admitted to hospital as a result of an episode of parasuicide is more commonly young, female, divorced,single or married, of low social class, living in an area of social deprivation and usually not psychiatrically ill.

These are statistical findings and there is a degree of overlap between the two. This is obvious if one considers that some patients classified as parasuicides are really failed suicides and some patients who kill themselves did not take their overdose with a definite intention of suicide. This highlights the difficulties in the categorical system used for classification in this area which places such a heavy weighting on lethality rather than

Table 15.1 Comparison of characteristics of suicides and parasuicides (UK)

	Parasuicide	Suicide
Incidence and recent trends	Now 20–30 times more common than suicide. Marked rise in incidence in last 20 years	Rate relatively steady; slight decline in England and Wales
Seasonal variation	None demonstrated	Peak in April, May
Age	Younger > older	Older > younger
Sex	Females > males	Males> females
Social class (males)	Lower > middle > upper	Upper > lower > middle
Marital status	Highest rates in divorced and single	Highest rates in divorced, single and widowed
Social isolation	Not associated	Associated
Urban/rural	Commoner in cities; associated ecologically with poverty	Commoner in cities; associated ecologically with social disorganization.
Employment status	Higher rates in unemployed	Higher rates in unemployed, retired
Method	Nearly all use self-poisoning; benzodiazepines and minor analgesics are commonest	Majority are self-poisoning; barbiturates are commonest. One third use more violent methods
Mental illness	Less strong association; depression is commonest	Strong association; depression is commonest
Alcohol and drug abuse	Association	Association
Personality	Sociopathic	Sociopathic,? Cyclothymic

Kreitman, N. and Dyer, J. A. T Suicide in relation to parasuicide. *Medicine Series No. 3*, **36**, 1827–1830. Medical Education (International) Ltd, Oxford.

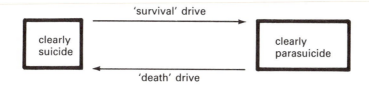

Figure 2 Motive in suicide/parasuicide

motive. With the individual in a clinical setting motive becomes paramount, but even then it may not be clear, as motive is often dimensional rather than categorical with many patients being ambivalent about whether they wish to live or die (see Figure 2).

SUICIDE AND PSYCHIATRIC ILLNESS

Many patients who commit suicide have consulted a doctor, either their general practitioner or a psychiatrist, in the weeks immediately prior to the act. Studies have suggested that most if not all of these patients were psychiatrically ill at the time of their suicide. The usual diagnoses are depression, alcoholism and personality disorder.

Depression

Manic-depressive illness and reactive depression carry a risk of suicide thirty times greater than that of the general population, and fifteen per cent of these patients will die by suicide. Risk factors include bereavement, a family history of suicide, a previous episode of attempted suicide, and ideas of guilt and worthlessness in the mental state. As depressive illnesses are potentially treatable it is mandatory that suicidal ideation is sought for in patients with this condition.

Alcoholism

Alcoholics have a particularly high suicide rate with a frequency of ten per cent of alcoholics in treatment and twenty per cent of known alcoholics. Old male alcoholics are most at risk particularly following loss of a spouse by bereavement or divorce or when the patient is depressed or has suffered physical damage.

Personality disorders

Patients with personality disorder may commit suicide either by design or by misjudgment during an act of parasuicide. In these cases warnings have often been given, and there may have been previous episodes of deliberate self-harm and a history of difficulties in coping with life such as a poor work record, unsatisfactory relationships and alcohol abuse. .

Other psychiatric illnesses

Some patients with psychotic illnesses may kill themselves while their judgement is impaired, as a response to paranoid delusions or hallucinations, though without the formed intent to commit suicide. An example of this is the patient with an acute confusional state who jumped out of a window because he thought the nurses were running after him to kill him. In these people the affect is predominantly one of anxiety rather than depression. Depression occurring as a reaction to any psychiatric or chronic physical illness may lead to suicide. Anorexia nervosa and epilepsy are also associated with a higher than average risk of suicide. Suicide may occur in schizophrenia as a result of a passivity phenomenon when the patient is compelled to kill himself.

SUICIDE IN CHILDREN

Suicide in children is no longer unheard of and tends to be associated with preceding suicidal behaviour often within the previous twenty-four hours, psychiatric illness in the child or family, or difficulties at home. In one study nearly half of the children who committed suicide did so using highly lethal methods.

SUICIDE AND HOMICIDE

In a number of cases of murder the murderer proceeds to commit suicide after committing his crime. This is particularly likely in situations where murder has occurred as part of a grief reaction due to the break-up of a relationship, but also occurs in depressive illnesses, particularly in the puerperium when the patient, deluded that a disaster is imminent, may kill her loved children in order to spare them suffering.

METHODS USED IN SUICIDE AND PARASUICIDE

Most people who commit acts of parasuicide take overdoses, usually of psychotropic drugs, especially benzodiazepines or analgesics obtainable across the counter. Not infrequently, alcohol is taken at the same time. For completed suicides the method most commonly used is still drug overdose, usually barbiturates, or other psychotropic drugs such as antidepressants and analgesics, but about one third, usually men, use more violent means including hanging, shooting, stabbing and precipitation.

INTENTIONS IN PARASUICIDE

Only a small number of parasuicides are failed suicides. In other cases motivation includes the following:

1 To obtain immediate relief from intolerable stress
2 To manipulate a situation; for example, to force an errant boyfriend or husband to modify his ways
3 In order to attract attention whether as part of a manipulative gesture or because of true distress which cannot be communicated in any other way — a 'cry for help'
4 As an aggressive act to make 'important' others feel guilty and anxious
5 In order to tempt fate without caring about the outcome.

Prognosis of parasuicide

Twenty to thirty per cent of patients who commit acts of parasuicide will repeat the act within twelve months. Predictive factors for repetition include alcohol and drug abuse, psychopathic personality disorder, previous parasuicide, past psychiatric history, residential mobility, unemployment, low social class and criminal record. One to two per cent of parasuicides will die from suicide in a one to two year follow up period, which is a rate about one hundred times greater than that of the general population. The more closely the parasuicide patient resembles the suicide patient profile, the greater is the risk of subsequent death by suicide; though in all cases the risk depends on the individual situation.

ASSESSMENT OF SUICIDE

It is mandatory that the risk of suicide is assessed in all patients with emotional disorders. There is no evidence that asking about suicidal ideation

Table 15.2 Assessment of the suicidal: some factors affecting the risk

1 Personal and social
M > F; aged over 40
Marital status: widowed, divorced or separated
Immigrant
Mode of living: alone, does not belong to a domestic group
Occupation: unoccupied or unemployed; works in recreational sevices; retired
District: socially disorganized urban areas; resort towns

2 Previous history
Family history of affective disorder, suicide, alcoholism
Previous history of affective disorder, alcoholism
Previous suicide attempt
Soon after onset; at the beginning of treatment; six months following discharge from active treatment

3 Life stresses
Bereavement and separations; moving house; loss of job
In alcoholics: domestic and social complications of drinking
Incapacitating terminal illness in elderly

4 Personality
Cyclothymic; sociopathic (impulsive, violent, capricious, delinquent)
Excessive drinking and drug dependency

5 Psychiatric illness
Depression, notably manic-depressive and recurrent depression
Alcoholism and other addictions
Early dementia and confusional states in elderly
Organic brain syndromes (epilepsy and head injury)
Combinations of the above

6 Symptoms
Depressive: persistent insomnia; dejected appearance, slowed speech, and loss of weight
Loss of usual interests, listlessness and social withdrawal
Hopelessness and pessimism
Ideas of unworthiness
Agitation and restlessness
Suicide thoughts
Alcoholics: medical and CNS complications

7 Circumstances of an attempt
Precautions taken against discovery
Preparatory acts: procuring means, affairs in order, warning statements; suicide note
Violent methods and more lethal drugs/poisons

Sainsbury, P. Suicide. *Medicine Series No. 1*, **30**, 1772–1776. Medical Education (International) Ltd, Oxford.

actually incites people to kill themselves, whereas failure to do so may lead to an otherwise preventable disaster. Patients should be asked how they view their future for example; whether it is bleak and hopeless or whether there is some light at the end of the tunnel. They may feel that they would like to go to sleep and not wake up, want to run away or escape, or would prefer to be dead. Suicidal ideation may be fleeting and unformed, may have been planned down to the last detail or even acted upon. Some suicidal patients are evasive, or insist that they could never kill themselves because of their family, religious beliefs or lack of courage. Where suicidal ideation is still suspected despite denial or excuses, it is worth asking the patient what he has to live for.

Important factors in the assessment of the risk of suicide are shown in Tables 15.2 and 15.3. Rating scales have been devised giving different ratings to some of these factors. Finally, the assessment is not complete until other informants have been interviewed; both to give an objective and possibly more honest account of symptoms, behaviour and ideation and to establish the support network in the person's environment.

Table 15.3 Circumstances of the act associated with suicidal intent

Isolation (no-one nearby)

Timing (so that intervention is unlikely)

Other precautions to avoid intervention or discovery (e.g. making excuses for not turning up where expected)

Not acting to get help after act

Final acts in anticipation of death (e.g. making a will, arranging insurance)

Active preparation for attempt (e.g. making special arrangements to obtain the means)

Suicide note

Adapted from Beck, A. T., Schuyler, D., and Herman, I. (1974). Development of suicidal intent scales in *The Prediction of Suicide* (Eds. Beck, A. T., Resnick, H. L. P. and Lettieri, D.); Bowie, Maryland: Charles Press.

Kreitman, N. and Dyer, J. A. T. Suicide in relation to parasuicide. *Medicine Series No. 3*, **36**, 1827–1830. Medical Education (International) Ltd, Oxford.

SELF-MUTILATION

In some societies self-mutilation is culturally normal and used for enhancing attractiveness, as a sign of status, to frighten enemies or as part of a religious rite. However, in this country self-mutilation is usually pathological, although even here cultural factors may be relevant. When the mutilation is due to psychological factors this may be as part of failed suicide, as a reaction to delusions or hallucinations, or most commonly as part of a personality disorder.

In the latter group self-mutilation usually takes the form of wrist-slashing, with the patient inflicting multiple lacerations on the wrists and arms and occasionally on other parts of the body, for example, the abdomen. It is commoner in women in late adolescence and the early twenties. There is no suicidal intent nor is it usually attention-seeking but occurs as a response to mounting tension and is associated with depersonalization and accompanied by a feeling of relief and satisfaction and the absence of pain. In some patients there is a compulsive or even orgasmic quality to the act. These patients often abuse alcohol and drugs, have sexual problems, disturbances of eating, a history of truancy and delinquency, a history of overdose, low self-esteem and poor self-image. It has been suggested that these patients often have links with the medical profession.

CASE HISTORY

ELIZABETH JENKINS

Elizabeth Jenkins, a 41-year-old housewife, was admitted in coma to an intensive care unit. She had been found by her husband unconscious in bed at home, with a polythene bag tied over her head. Upon rescuscitation she recovered consciousness but was confused and showed signs of cerebral irritation over the next forty-eight hours. She remained uncooperative and relatively mute and the following history was obtained largely from her family and partly, later from her.

Mrs Jenkins had been married for eighteen years, and had four children; sons aged 16 and 7 and daughters aged 14 and 11 years. Two years before she had had a hysterectomy for menor-rhagia and although she had appeared to have recovered thoroughly, her husband described a gradual change in personality beginning a few months after the operation. She had previously been cheerful, competent, uncomplaining and supportive and was an excellent home-maker and mother. Over the last eighteen months or so she had become gradually less interested in the family, had been withdrawn, unhappy and irritable. She was bitter and angry about the operation, of which she had been frightened, and recently had become quite remote from her husband, both physically and emotionally. She maintained practical care of the children but was no longer openly affectionate. During the last year, her mother, to whom she had not been close and who intimidated Elizabeth, had become ill, with increasing dependence and demands for care and support from the family.

Mr and Mrs Jenkins had met at teacher training college and become engaged shortly after qualifi-cation. After their marriage Mr Jenkins had begun training for the ministry and was subsequently ordained; Mrs Jenkins supported him in his vo-cation although her religious beliefs were never as intense as his. They had planned and welcomed a large family despite their low income, which Mrs Jenkins had, on occasion, supplemented by teaching. Five years ago, the Reverend Mr Jenkins had obtained a parish in a small country town; his wife had worked hard maintaining the large, cold vicarage and helped him with his parish duties. She had not complained of ill health until she collapsed one day from anaemia due to menorrhagia.

Her husband took his pastoral duties very seriously, was always available to his parishioners and was a tireless worker. He had always believed that his wife shared his views and was happy to have an open door to all comers. He had been hurt and shocked when in recent months she had refused to organize functions and support parish work, and had stopped attending church. He felt betrayed and unsupported and for the first time in their marriage the couple began to have rows. In the course of these, Mrs Jenkins accused her husband of caring more for his parishioners than for herself and said that he would only realize his need of her if she were not there. Her husband tended to ignore these remarks, feeling that they were patently untrue so she could not really have meant them.

The attempt at suicide took place on a Sunday morning when the family were at church. Mrs Jenkins was still in bed when they left, saying she had slept poorly the previous night and did not feel well. She took a handful of (benzodiazepine) sleeping tablets prescribed by her GP, locked herself in her bedroom, and tied a polythene bag round her head with the cord from her husband's dressing gown. Her husband had returned from conducting the service, found the bedroom door locked from the inside and, with help from a neighbour, had broken the door down to find his wife blue and unconscious.

Psychiatric assessment of Mrs Jenkins some seventy-two hours after her admission added little information. She appeared retarded, and refused to talk about the attempt at suicide, shrugging her shoulders and saying only that she would not do it again.

Questions

What factors indicate the seriousness or other-wise of this attempted suicide? Could it have been foreseen?

The assessment of the risk of suicide in this case should concentrate on these areas: the previous history of the patient, the circumstances of the attempt and the mental state and current suicidal ideation on assessment after the attempt.

At first sight, Mrs Jenkins is not in a high risk category either for suicide or for attempted suicide. She has no past history or family history of any psychiatric illness or previous attempted suicide, has no physical illness, is in a stable marriage, is not socially isolated and has no prob-lems with alcohol. There is, however, clear evidence of developing depression over a relatively long period, together with estrangement from her family. There is insufficient evidence at this point to decide the type or severity of the depressive condition.

The circumstances of the act are also somewhat mixed in their predictive value. Mrs Jenkins attempted suicide in a dramatic and relatively unusual way, and by locking the door took pains against premature discovery and very nearly died. These factors indicate a very serious attempt. Set against this, however, is her knowledge of the time the family would return from a routine engagement, and the overt, possibly manipulative hostility demonstrated to her husband by the timing of the attempt and the use of his clothing to aid it. Since Mrs Jenkins will not at this point discuss the attempt, one cannot say that her suicidal intent was low; indeed, her silence indicates the likelihood that it was high. Her mental state is abnormal and indicates either a depressive stupor or a hostile refusal to co-operate. Post-anoxic brain damage has not yet been excluded and it must be borne in mind that Mrs Jenkins has a history of fear and dislike of hospital treatment.

It is, however, the fact this behaviour is so out of character with Mrs Jenkins' previous personality which demonstrates its seriousness. She does not make histrionic gestures and therefore the likelihood that this is one which has gone wrong is extremely low. She must be considered as presenting a major suicide risk.

Could this attempt have been foreseen or prevented? She was visiting her GP with complaints of sleeplessness, and a sympathetic GP who knew her well might have been able to understand the significance of her changed personality, but it is likely that an unassertive, uncomplaining woman did not find it easy to divulge her state of mind to her doctor because of her shame and fear of failure. She undoubtedly had tried to tell her husband of her despair, but his own psychopathology prevented him from hearing it; he had a view of his wife as coping and compliant which was not readjusted by the reality of her condition and he was preoccupied with his extra family responsibilities. In addition, the insidious, slow onset of her change in behaviour acted against an awareness that a very serious change was taking place.

This case demonstrates the difficulty of a true assessment of people who are seen by themselves and others as competent 'givers'. They find it difficult to accept that they need help, and hide their feelings of increasing despair. When this is a feature of a whole family's way of life, as in this case, early intervention and treatment are often precluded.

16

Excitement states

The term excitement is used to describe states of agitation, overactivity over-talkativeness, irritability, or undue exhilaration. It is important to distinguish between organic and functional causes. This depends partly upon recognizing the syndrome: for instance mania, or acute confusional state; and partly upon careful elicitation of the history for aetiological factors, such as heredity, personality, drugs, and physical illness.

MANIA

The manic syndrome is one of the most clearly defined in psychiatry, but the diagnosis is frequently missed. Table 16.1 shows the diagnostic criteria for mania according to DSM–III.

The criterion of duration, though useful for research purposes, may be too rigid clinically, particularly since hospitalization may be an administrative as much as a clinical decision.

The elevation of mood is usually described by the patient in terms such as 'on top of the world', 'never felt better', or 'extremely fit'. It may be accompanied by a sense of religious revelation. Sometimes the mood seems fatuous but often there is an infectious quality to the good humour which cheers other people and leads to laughter. However, the sustained elation is wearing on those around the patient. Any frustration of his ambitious plans provokes anger and a sense of persecution which may lead to abuse and aggression. Tearful swings of mood occur, especially when the patient is confronted with personal problems. The swings of depression or hostility tend to last only a minute or so, but in some cases the irritability or depression can effec-

Table 16.1 Mania: Diagnostic criteria (DSM–III)

1 Mood: elated or irritable

plus

2 Three of the following:
overactivity
increased talkativeness or pressure of speech
flight of ideas or racing thoughts
distractibility
grandiosity (including grandiose delusions)
indiscreet behaviour with poor judgment
decreased sleep

plus

3 Duration: More than one week or any duration if hospitalized

tively mask the elation for longer. In some patients the admixture of depression and elation may be so marked as to lead to the diagnosis of a mixed affective state (see below).

Overactivity is apparent in an excessive use of gestures and the patient's tendency to leave the chair during the interview. Sometimes this excessive energy is used effectively but more often actions are hurried and clumsy. Speech may be characterized by an increase in rate (pressure of speech) and it may be difficult to interrupt the patient. The voice is often raised and this may lead to hoarseness.

In flight of ideas the associations of thoughts proceed in a fast and lively but usually understandable way, and puns and other sorts of wordplay are common (see Chapter 11). The patient's thoughts are easily distracted by changes in his surroundings. Distractibility may lead to forget-fulness, with suspiciousness; for example, that others are taking his belongings. He may react to this by gathering his possessions together.

The manic patient may be grandiose, with high self-esteem and ambitiousness. He may have delusions of wealth or of royal descent. Female patients may falsely believe that they are pregnant. Caution must be exercised before diagnosing such beliefs as delusional, since sexual promiscuity is common in this group. Other indiscreet behaviour includes disinhibition and over-familiarity, and over-spending which may be domestic, as with the patient who buys one thousand crates of apples. There is a decreased need for sleep, with the patient awakening from a short sleep feeling energetic. Although appetites are increased or disinhibited, distractibility tends to preclude satisfaction.

Differential Diagnosis

The presence of paranoid or grandiose delusions or of auditory hallucinations, both of which may occur in mania, may lead to the misdiagnosis of schizophrenia. Auditory hallucinations in mania occur in the form of voices addressing the patient, with a content which is reassuring or exciting to the patient. Some patients when manic drink more alcohol than usual in an attempt to relax or to enjoy themselves; this can obscure the underlying mania.

Histrionic behaviour may lead to the diagnosis of personality disorder and hysterical dissociation to hysterical neurosis, while the diagnosis of mania is missed. The less floridly disturbed patient may not be recognized as ill at all, until, perhaps, he has been arrested for an offence which arose from his symptoms. Even then the correct diagnosis may be delayed.

Because mania is often improved within a few days by antipsychotic medication, more importance should be given to the history than to the present mental state when assessing patients who have recently received such medication for excitement states.

Some patients with symptoms fulfilling the inclusion criteria for diagnosing mania have in addition one or more of the 'first rank symptoms' of schizophrenia described by Schneider (see Chapter 17, Table 17.6). Disagreement can arise about diagnosis. According to the Research Diagnostic Criteria, the diagnosis is 'schizoaffective disorder' (schizomania). According to DSM–III the diagnosis is 'mania with psychotic features' if the content of the delusions or hallucinations is congruent with raised mood; otherwise the diagnosis is 'mania with mood-incongruent psychotic features'. Catatonic symptoms (e.g. stereotypies, posturing, negativism, mutism, stupor) may occur in mania; according to the DSM–III such patients have 'mania with mood-incongruent psychotic features'. Mania should not be diagnosed if these psychotic features are present before the manic syndrome has developed, or after it has remitted; such patients have schizoaffective disorder according to the DSM-III.

Occasionally, manic patients become disorientated, or have other symptoms suggestive of a confusional state, including visual hallucinations. These are more likely to occur in severe cases and where self- neglect and physical exhaustion have developed. Evidence of chest infection and cardiac failure should be sought. 'Delirious mania' is a term used for cases with confusional symptoms without evidence of underlying physical illness.

Mania illness occurs with the usual frequency in persons with mental retardation. In the severely mentally retarded the diagnosis may be less obvious, but can be made on the basis of the cyclical nature of the disorder, the changes in mood, activity and sleep and the family history. A different excitement state may arise in subnormal persons who react to severe stress with a state of chaotic restlessness.

Manic illness in certain groups is particularly likely to be misdiagnosed as schizophrenia. Thus mania occurring in adolescence tends to have a higher incidence of psychotic features. This is important since although the mean age of this first episode of bipolar manic-depressive disorder is about thirty years, the most common age of true onset is between fifteen and nineteen years.

Cultural factors may alter the manifestations of mania and create diagnostic difficulties. For example in a conservative Protestant sect some of the manifestations of mania (overspending, disinhibition and grandiosity) may conflict with the prevailing religious values (frugality, sexual discretion, and the sign of pride). Selfconsciousness and embarrassment about his euphoria can make the manic person seem affectively incongruous. Racial differences in the incidence of manic illness are probably more apparent than real. For instance, China, Nigeria and Denmark all have similar incidences of mania with similar clinical presentations. In Nigeria, fewer cases are associated with depressive episodes and there is more recurrent unipolar mania. Patients of Caribbean origin often present with religiosity that may be delusional. Some of these seem to be acute paranoid reactions to recent or chronic stress; others may be more appropriately diagnosed as mania.

The History

Manic illness is usually associated with a history of depressive episodes and therefore can be recognized as part of a 'bipolar' manic-depressive disorder. Some patients have recurrent 'unipolar' mania but the distinction between unipolar and bipolar mania has not yet been shown to be useful. In contrast with schizophrenic patients, bipolar patients show a slight predominance of higher socioeconomic class and educational and occupational attainment. Manic episodes are very disruptive to all areas of the patient's life and there is an increased rate of divorce, although the majority of marriages stabilize on the patient's recovery. The phenomenon of 'assortative mating' occurs in bipolar illness: patients tend to choose for a marriage partner someone with a personal or family history indicative of predisposition to the same condition.

The blood relatives of manic patients have a greatly increased risk of developing mania. The risk round in first degree relatives is about ten per cent compared to about 0.7% of the general population. Relatives also have an increased risk of depressive illness without manic episodes.

In the few months before admission to hospital with mania, patients may well have experienced more than the usual number of undesirable life-events (of a kind unlikely to have been a result of the illness). The events that most obviously precede manic illnesses are bereavements and personal separations. Work-related problems and loss of role are also significant.

Since mania is one of the most insightless forms of psychiatric disorder, information from independent informants is essential in determining the premorbid personality of the patient. Prominent mood traits (hyperthymia, cyclothymia, or depressive traits) are commonly described. An association with pyknic build has been suggested.

Secondary Mania

A manic state may develop following a clear physical disturbance by drugs or by disease or in the puerperium. When this occurs in a patient without a past or family history of affective disorder, the term 'secondary mania' is used. These manic syndromes occur in clear consciousness and are therefore distinguised from acute confusional states. Table 16.2 shows the factors that have been associated with secondary mania. Some of these can also produce excitement states which differ from true mania, and are discussed below.

Table 16.2 Secondary mania

Drugs/medication
 corticosteroids
 L-dopa
 MAOI's — isoniazid
 dopamine agonists (bromocriptine etc)
 thyroid hormones

Psychostimulants
 amphetamines
 cocaine
 cannabis
 alcohol
 anticholinergics (procyclidine, benzhexol)

Metabolic disorders
 thyrotoxicosis
 porphyria

Organic brain disease
 dementia
 temporal lobe epilepsy
 neoplasm
 neurosyphilis
 multiple sclerosis.

Intoxications

Both amphetamines and cannabis may, in large doses or in susceptible individuals, poduce a state resembling mania. However, both may also produce a paranoid psychosis almost indistinguishable from acute schizophrenia. Screening of the urine for these drugs is very important in the assessment of new patients with excitement states, and of patients whose condition suddenly deteriorates for no apparent cause, when they may have had access to drugs. The physical signs of amphetamine intoxication include dilated pupils and raised blood pressure. There may also be needle marks over veins. Cannabis intoxication is associated with conjuctival inflammation.

Pathological intoxication (mania à potu)

Pathological intoxication is an idiosyncratic reaction to alcohol in persons predisposed by brain damage or by abnormal personality. An abrupt deterioration in behaviour occurs after drinking alcohol. The degree of excitement may be extraordinarily severe with senseless aggressive behaviour and assault. The period of excitement is followed by sleep, and subsequent amnesia. Although the person may not appear the worse for drink, blood alcohol levels may be very high during the episode. Abnormalities of the EEG are common on recovery. Hypoglycaemia may be a contributory factor in the attack.

Anticholinergics

Certain anticholinergic drugs, particularly procylidine and benzhexol, have psychostimulant effects, and are sometimes abused. Although large doses are most often found to produce a toxic-confusional state with visual hallucinations, a state resembling mania in clear consciousness has also been described. Dilated pupils and dry mouth are suggestive physical signs.

Thyroid hormones

Hyperactivity and irritability are common symptoms in thyrotoxicosis but the main diagnostic similarity is not with mania but with anxiety neurosis. The commencement of treatment of myxoedema with thyroid hormones leads in some cases to the worsening of psychotic symptoms, and the emergence of a state resembling mania.

The occurrence of thyrotoxicosis in a patient with a history of bipolar affective disorder can lead to the development of a manic state.

NEUROSYPHILIS

This is now a rare but partly treatable disease. It may present with the insidious onset of an expansive and euphoric state with grandiose delusions, resembling mania. Alternatively the patient may be paranoid and agitated. Physical examination may reveal tabetic facies, Argyll-Robertson pupils, tremor, dysarthria, ataxia, spasticity, absent ankle jerks, extensor plantar reflexes, absent vibration sensitivity, and evidence of dementia. Serological tests and the immunological reaction and cell count of the cerebrospinal fluid (CSF) confirm the diagnosis.

DEMENTIA

In the early states of dementia of Alzheimer's type, affective symptoms, especially agitation, are common. The disturbances may be episodic and include a state resembling mania, with or without paranoid delusions. Careful examination and history-taking will reveal an insidious onset with deterioration in personality and memory. Specific deficits in higher cerebral functions, such as dysphasia and dyspraxia, may be detected. Helpful investigations include psychometric testing, EEG and CAT scan.

EPILEPSY

Irritability, tension and depression are sometimes present for several days or weeks in the prodrome of an epileptic convulsion. During a temporal lobe seizure (complex partial seizure) there may be a period of 'automatism' associated with irritability, fear, and bizarre, often stereotyped, behaviour, which may rarely be dangerous. Usually such automatisms last only a few minutes or less and are associated with dense amnesia for the episode. After a generalized convulsion there may be a post-ictal confusional state, in which the patient reacts angrily to interference. Goal-directed aggressive behaviour or criminal behaviour is unusual at this time, but senseless violence may occur. Syndromes resembling mania or delirious mania have been associated with the inter-ictal state in patients who have had temporal lobe epilepsy for several years. In assessing patients who have recovered from a brief mania-like episode it is therefore important to look for evidence of epileptic phenomena (see Chapter 20).

ORGANIC CONFUSIONAL STATES

An organic confusional state may present with symptoms of 'excitement', including irritability, restlessness, noisiness, over-sensitivity to stimuli, and emotional lability. Whether these symptoms predominate depends upon the patient's personality, and upon the cause of the organic syndrome. Excitement states are especially likely to be associated with drug-intoxication, withdrawal of alcohol or sedatives (delirium tremens), and with hypoglycaemia. Pointers towards an organic cause of an excitement state include disorientation in time and place, fluctuations in degree of impairment with increased confusion and agitation at night, and visual illusions and hallucinations. Subsequent amnesia may be indicative of an organic basis for a reported episode of excitement.

PARANOID STATES

Paranoid states may be associated with excitement in the form of anger and pressure of speech. However, the central abnormality is the distortion of beliefs concerning the patient's relationships with other people. The distinction from mania on the basis of the mental state is occasionally difficult, but there is usually no elation, there is over-inclusive thinking rather than flight of ideas, and there are not the characteristic changes in sleep and appetites. In paranoid reactions the history may reveal a paranoid personality type and an obvious stress associated with the onset of illness. In paranoid schizophrenia the patient may respond to auditory hallucinations of an abusive or threatening kind by being angry and vociferous.

CATATONIC EXCITEMENT AND SCHIZOPHRENIA

Excitement states may occur in the course of schizophrenia, usually in cases associated also with catatonic symptoms. As discussed in Chapter 3, 'catatonic' symptoms may occur in a variety of functional and organic disorders. The term 'catatonic excitement' is best applied to cases where it alternates with a catatonic stupor. The excitement takes the form of restlessness with reckless, impulsive and aimless actions, often of a very peculiar kind; for instance during a catatonic excitement a young woman ran into a shop in central London wearing only in girdle and carried out a colour television set. The mood is elated or irritable, but prone to astonishing changes, with depression and hostility, and there may be a 'deadpan' facial expression.

There is a particular type of disorder of thought form with neologisms, contrived expressions, or talking past the point, *vorbeireden*. Severe cases show verbigeration. There may be extreme sexual excitement and open masturbation. The condition tends to deteriorate during menstruation. Although difficulty may sometimes arise in differentiating catatonic excitement from mania, the senselessness of the activity contrasts with the purposefulness of activity in the mania patient; the remoteness and unattractive quality of the hilarity contrast with the infectious quality of mania. Many of the symptoms of catatonia can be formulated as a disorder of volition; during excitement, the patient seems to follow whatever impulse arises in him. Hallucinations and delusions occur, but may be difficult to elicit.

REACTIVE EXCITEMENT

It has long been recognized that psychotic states may follow extreme degrees of stress. The symptoms and signs may be indistinguishable from those in the functional psychoses, and the diagnosis may only become clear from the natural history of the disorder. Such conditions classically remit upon removal of the stress without other specific treatment. This is given added significance by the fact that stress is a common precipitant of functional psychosis and indeed its presence is regarded as a good prognostic pointer in schizophrenia. In addition drug-induced psychosis may present a similar clinical picture with remission after the removal of the drug. It is clear that diagnostic and terminological pitfalls abound in this area.

Since the content of psychotic phenomena is influenced by culture, diagnostic difficulties are especially likely to arise when the therapist and patient come from different cultures. The situation is further complicated in the presence of a language barrier. Certain personalities are particularly predisposed to develop psychoses under stress (borderline personalities). In addition to mimicking the functional psychoses the mental state may contain a bizarre admixture of abnormal phenomena.

These conditions have been given many labels including reactive excitement, schizophreniform disorder, psychogenic psychosis, and hysterical psychosis. In ICD–9 they are included in the category 298.0–298.8 (other non-organic psychoses; see Chapter 17).

ANXIETY-ELATION PSYCHOSIS

This is one of the forms of 'cycloid psychosis', a diagnostic group recognized especially by Scandinavian psychiatrists. In anxiety-elation psychosis, the patient shows mood swings between depression or anxiety, and elation or ecstasy. Psychotic episodes also include delusions or hallucinations. The prognosis resembles that of manic-depressive illness more closely than that of schizophrenia, but the recurrence rate may be higher and the premorbid personality may show more neurotic traits. The value of this diagnostic category has yet to be established in other countries, whose diagnostic systems would regard these patients as having either schizoaffective or mixed-affective psychosis, or schizophrenia.

'Motility psychosis' is another form of cycloid psychosis, in which motor aspects of mania predominate with clowning movements and over-activity, but not pressure of speech.

AGITATED DEPRESSION

The agitation of some depressed patients may be so severe as to dominate the presentation. The patient appears restless and impatient, wringing his hands, picking at his face or hair, and unable to settle in a chair or in a room. He may ask questions repetitively in an anxious and importuning manner, or reiterate depressive statements such as 'I will never get better'. The painful quality of the affect and the morbid content of the talk reveal the depressive nature of the underlying disorder.

FRONTAL LOBE SYNDROME

Lesions affecting the frontal lobes may produce a syndrome of fatuous euphoria, disinhibition, and over-talkativeness, accompanied by outbursts of irritability and childish excitement. A lack of foresight and loss of finesse, lead to indiscreet behaviour. Frontal lobe lesions tend to be 'silent' in the sense that intellectual performance is not obviously impaired. Slow-growing frontal tumours (e.g. meningiomas) may remain undiagnosed for many years since physical signs are relatively scarce. Amongst the most important is the grasp reflex, and optic atrophy and anosmia may be secondary features.

HISTRIONIC AND EXPLOSIVE PERSONALITY DISORDER

Histrionic personalities are inclined to excessive and exaggerated displays of emotion. Explosive personalities cannot control their emotions, and are liable to unrestrained displays of anger in response to mild annoyances. These habitual shows of emotion are short-lived compared with the conditions described above.

MIXED AFFECTIVE STATES

This term is used to describe the coexistence of manic and depressive symptomatology. Mania and depression involve changes in mood, activity and thinking, and these three areas of functioning can vary independently to produce mixed states. The commonest situation in which this occurs is during the onset of mania or during a change over of 'switch' between mania and depression. However, in some patients a mixed state may develop and recover without a pure depression or mania emerging. Theoretically six possible permutations could occur. The best recognized is manic stupor, in which the patient has extreme psychomotor retardation but appears elated and later describes having experienced racing thoughts. Depression with flight of ideas is also recognized. In addition the vegetative symptoms of depression, such as anorexia, may accompany mania. If one further allows that the thought content may vary (so that hypochondriacal ideas may accompany elation and grandiosity may occur in depression), the area becomes very complicated; it is possible that some patients who would be diagnosed as having mania with mood-incongruent delusions might be better regarded as having a mixed affective disorder. Since transient depression of mood is very common in mania, the term 'mixed affective state' is best reserved for cases in which syndromes of depression and mania are both present sufficiently to meet the diagnostic criteria according to DSM–III).

CASE HISTORY

BRIAN HARPER

Mr Brian Harper was a 25-year-old Jamaican clerk who was brought to the local casualty department by the police, having smashed a window in the High Street. When apprehended he had behaved peculiarly, talked non-stop and appeared very excitable. When examined by the duty psychiatrist, Mr Harper was irritable and agitated, showed great pressure of speech with flight of ideas and delusions of grandeur. He refused to accept that there was anything wrong with him and was so resistant to being admitted to hospital that four male nurses were required to restrain him sufficiently for intramuscular sedation to be given.

His girlfriend, Camilla, was contacted and she gave the following story. Brian had been relatively well up to forty-eight hours prior to his admission. He had held down a good job as a clerk in an insurance company where he was well liked and highly thought of. The couple had known each other for seven years and had lived together for the last five. Initially they had been happy without any major rows. However, in the last six months, Brian had started drinking heavily and Camilla had formed a friendship with a male colleague at work. After a series of increasingly violent arguments, she had decided to leave Brian, and had communicated her decision to him the previous week, saying that she would leave immediately. Brian had begged her to stay and she agreed, reluctantly, to do so. However, two days before his admission, they had a blazing row which ended in his hitting her. Camilla then walked out; she returned five hours later to collect her clothes.

On the following day, she was phoned by a neighbour who was worried because Brian had been shouting all night, and had kept the stereo on at full volume. Camilla did not return to the flat and was phoned again the next day with a similar story. When the neighbour threatened to call the police unless Brian quietened down, she took pity on him and went to the flat, taking her new boyfriend with her for protection. On entering the flat, she was greeted by a scence of devastation: all the furniture was smashed, clothes were strewn all over the place and hers were ripped up, while in the bedroom there were three empty whisky bottles and a number of empty beer cans. There was no sign of Brian and she did not see him again until she visited the hospital subsequent to his admission.

When pressed about the details of his behaviour and emotional state in the weeks prior to their break-up, Camilla said that he had been drinking more heavily than usual, had been sleeping poorly and had become increasingly irritable. He was talking a lot, but his speech did not always make sense. He had spent quite large sums of money buying clothes he did not really need. She believed there was no past or family psychiatric history, and this was later confirmed by Brian.

When Brian became able to give a coherent account of himself, he said that his parents had come over to England in the early 1950s and he had been born here. His early childhood was unremarkable, but there had been some trouble at secondary school with truancy and rudeness to the teachers, although this was not markedly different from the behaviour of his peers. He had been happy at home where the atmosphere was described as warm.

After leaving school at the age of sixteen, he went to college for a year and studied office management. Following this, he worked in an estate agent's office for two years until it closed down and he was made redundant. He was only out of work for three weeks before finding his present job, where he had been for the last six years. Brian agreed with Camilla's assessment of their relationship, and confirmed that he had been drinking more alcohol in the months prior to the admission. He also admitted that he had, of late, been abusing drugs, mainly cannabis. He was unable to shed any more light on the events of the forty-eight hours leading up to his admission.

Questions

What are the possible diagnoses?
How can the diagnosis be clarified following admission to hospital?

The overactivity, pressure of speech, flight of ideas, delusions of grandeur and lack of insight are consistent with the diagnosis of mania. This is supported by Camilla's account of increasing irritability, overspending, garrulousness, sleeplessness and possibly increased drinking in the weeks leading up to his admission. Absence of a past or family history of manic-depressive illness does not rule out this out.

An alternative diagnosis is of a stress-induced reactive excitement; other non-organic psychoses — excitative type (ICD–9 298.1); the stress in this case being the break-up of the relationship. It is suggested that this diagnosis is especially common in the West Indian immigrant population. It is possible to consider Brian's increased drinking and spending as ways of coping with the increased stress, the latter in a similar way to comfort eating. Sleep impairment may be merely an outward sign of an increased level of arousal as may irritability and garrulousness. The negative

past and family history of an affective illness lends some support to this diagnosis.

It may be extraordinarily difficult in these cases to differentiate between mania and stress-induced reactive excitement, especially given the research findings of an increase in life events prior to the onset of an episode of mania. The diagnosis may only become apparent in retrospect, either from the pattern of response to treatment or following the occurrence of further similar disorders.

Alcohol and drugs, both of which we know Brian has been abusing, may lead to states of excitement and, in all such cases, evidence of abuse should be rigorously sought with details of type, quantity, frequency and duration of substance abuse. Such abuse leads either to brief episodes of disturbed behaviour with abnormalities in the mental state which remit after cessation of abuse or after the withdrawal period; or in some cases to a longer lasting paranoid psychosis.

Patients with acute confusional states may behave bizarrely and violently as may those with catatonic excitement, but these conditions would only account for the acute outburst. On the other hand, it may be that this entire period of disturbance merely represents the demonstration of extreme anger, not pathological in nature or degree. It is very important not to confuse anger and mania, which may present difficulties in transcultural settings. Finally, the differential diagnosis of explosive outbursts must always include personality disorder, but in Brian's case there is no evidence of this. In addition, the presence of delusions of grandeur and flight of ideas makes anger or personality disturbance alone much less likely than a psychotic illness.

On admission, a detailed mental state and physical examination must be carried out as far as the patient's co-operation will permit, to look in particular, for signs of mania, catatonia or acute organic confusion. Laboratory investigations include screening for drug and alcohol abuse and for physical illness. An EEG will help in the diagnosis of acute confusional states.

Until the diagnosis is clear, the patient should as far as possible, be left unsedated, in order not to mask vital diagnostic signs. In addition to the history already obtained, information about personality and past and present history should be gathered from relevant informants. Ward behaviour should be observed carefully, and an abreaction may be helpful if reactive excitement is suspected as the diagnosis. If the diagnosis remains unclear, and Brian's condition does not improve, a trial of major tranquillizers should follow. However, it must be remembered that this treatment is effective for all conditions of high arousal, including mania.

17

Strange ideas

It is useful to distinguish between the *form* and the *content* of abnormal ideas. The form refers to whether the idea is, for instance, an obsession, delusion, overvalued idea or example of thought insertion (see Table 17.1). The content refers to the theme of the idea, particularly as it concerns the person's relationship with others, and whether it is in keeping with the prevailing mood. The distinction between form and content is particularly important when cultural factors seem to influence symptoms. For example, a person brought up to believe in witchcraft may understandably account for alterations in his mood or physical wellbeing in such terms, but if he is convinced that a witch is using special powers to make him, and him alone, think thoughts that are not his own, he has a delusion of thought insertion, which carries the same diagnostic significance in all cultures. The cultural background helps in understanding the content of the delusion but does not explain the presence of a first rank symptom of schizophrenia.

Delusions are false beliefs; they may coincidentally be true, but it is the logical basis from which the belief is derived that is at fault. For example, a man may believe that he is being observed by the police, basing his belief on his observation that yellow minicars are parked at the corner of the street and that the assistant at the corner shop picked up the wrong newspaper when he went to buy one. It may be true that the police are observing him but neither of these two factors would normally be taken as evidence for this conclusion. Therefore whatever the ultimate truth of his situation his beliefs are delusional.

Sometimes during the onset or recovery from illness, the delusional belief is less firmly held and the patient may be persuaded at times that the belief is mistaken. This is called a 'partial delusion'.

Overvalued ideas are held with less conviction than delusions but tend to dominate the person's life and to be expressed with intense feeling. Their development is sometimes a consequence of

Table 17.1 Different forms of abnormal ideas

Delusion	A belief, inconsistent with the available information and not shared by others of the same cultural group, which is firmly held and cannot be dispelled by argument or proof to the contrary
Overvalued ideas	Deeply-held personal convictions that take precedence over all other ideas and may be understandable when the person's background is known
Ideas of reference	Occur in selfconscious individuals who feel that people take notice of them in a special way, or that events have a special significance for them, but realize that this feeling is a reflection of their own sensitivity
Obsession	An unpleasant content of consciousness which recurs or persists although it seems senseless to the individual, who tries strongly to stop it. It may be an idea, a mental image of fear or an impulse, and the content is usually of a sexual, aggressive or blasphemous kind
Confabulation	Plausible but inaccurate statements, such as occur in Korsakov's syndrome when they seem to fill gaps in the memory. This term should only be used when false ideas are directely due to cognitive deficit

affective illness and the belief may lose its supremacy after the mood has returned to normal. In other cases the overvalued ideas seem to arise from the person's experiences and continue thereafter to dominate his life.

Confabulation occur in Korsakov's syndrome (see Chapter 19). A similar phenomenon may be seen in pathological liars (pseudologia fantastica) when it is sometimes difficult to know whether the patient himself believes the ideas, which are often expressed in a convincing way. Occasionally insight is evident from the steps taken to persuade others, as in the case of a woman on remand for fraud who claimed to be pregnant with twins and used another patient's urine to obtain a positive pregnancy test. Some cases are best regarded as hysterical dissociative states. Such patients are seen in city casualty departments, repeatedly seeking admission to hospital and treatment for physical or psychiatric symptoms. They may exaggerate or simulate the physical signs, and usually discharge themselves when their deceit is discovered, only to present in another hospital (Munchausen's syndrome; chronic factitious disorders — DSM–III). Malingering differs from factitious disorder by the presence of an obviously recognizable and understandable goal that is pursued by the malingerer. In factitious disorder the goal is only understandable in terms of the subject's need to assume the role of a patient.

DIFFERENT FORMS OF DELUSIONS
(Table 17.2)

It is important to distinguish between delusions that arise suddenly with no understandable

Table 17.2 Different forms of delusion

Primary delusions
    Delusional mood
    Sudden delusional idea ('autochthonous delusion')
    Delusional perception

Secondary delusions
    e.g. Delusional misinterpretation

Shared delusions

Monosymptomatic delusions

connection to what has gone before (primary delusions) and those that develop secondary to an underlying abnormal mental state (secondary delusions). Secondarily delusions have some understandable connection between their content and the abnormal state from which they arose (e.g. mood-congruent delusions in depressive illness). Primary delusions are usually followed by a secondary delusional system.

Primary delusional experiences (delusional mood, sudden delusional idea and delusional perception) are almost diagnostic of the onset of schizophrenia. A delusional mood is a conviction that something is going on around the person which concerns him, but he does not know what it is. This may continue for some time before the patient develops a sudden delusional idea or a delusional perception. Sudden delusional ideas (autochthonous delusions) occur suddenly and fully formed in the patient's mind. In a delusional perception the patient attaches new meaning to a normal perception, and the delusional content cannot be understood as arising from the previous affective state or attitudes. For example a man who has been feeling uneasy for some days is cycling past a school, after seeing the gate he suddenly becomes convinced that all the children in the school are being locked in and tortured. By contrast delusional misinterpretation occurs when the patient's pre-existing disorder leads him to attach a delusional meaning to a perception; a manic patient who thinks he is assisting the police sees fishermen coming ashore each night and believes he is observing an invasion by the Russians; a depressive patient sees a spot on his skin and concludes that he has cancer; a paranoid patient sees car lights passing outside and believes that spies are passing messages about him. These are all secondary delusions based on misinterpretation in keeping with the patient's prevailing mood and attitudes.

In induced psychosis — shared paranoid disorder (usually folie à deux) — the delusion develops during a close relationship with another person who is already affected by a condition with delusions. The victim is usually highly impressionable (either through low intelligence or dependence upon the other person), and will gradually lose the abnormal beliefs when separated from his deluded associate.

Monosymptomatic delusions are delusions with a single theme, that are not secondary to another psychiatric illness, and are sustained over a considerable period without the development of other delusions, or personality change. In monosymptomatic hypochondriacal psychosis the patient has a delusional belief that he is affected by a disease of a single kind; a common symptom is the delusion of skin infestation, or of internal parasitosis or worms. Other monosymptomatic delusions that seem closely related to this are dysmorphophobic delusions (a conviction of personal ugliness or misshapenness — especially of face or sexual characteristics — despite evidence to the contarary), and olfactory delusions when the patient is convinced that he emits a foul smell. Such patients tend energetically to seek medical rather than psychological help and have a suicide risk. Longstanding cases of delusional hypochondriasis may lead to shared delusions (folie à deux). The condition may be regarded as a variant of paranoia and akin to monosymptomatic forms of delusions of infidelity (morbid jealousy), and erotomania (de Clerambault's syndrome).

DIFFERENT CONTENT OF DELUSIONS
(see Table 17.3)

Paranoid delusions

The term paranoid was originally used to describe any type of delusional condition. Nowadays it is most commonly used to refer to persecutory delusions. Delusions of persecution may arise as primary delusional experiences or may be secondary to hallucinations or passivity experiences, or arise in depressed or manic patients (see Chapters 14, 16, 18). Sources of persecution vary from organizations, such as the police, to individual acquaintances. If the subject makes his ideas known, it is not surprising that there may eventually come to be an element of truth in the persecutory ideas. Persecutory delusions may have a grandiose or depressive colouring: for example, a patient may believe that he is persecuted because of some special attribute such as wealth or royal descent which provokes jealousy. A persecutory quality is often a feature of other delusions.

Table 17.3 Content of delusions

Paranoid delusions (persecutory)
Delusions of control
Delusions of reference
Religious delusions
Delusions of infidelity
Delusions of love
Grandiose delusions

Depressive delusions
    guilt
    poverty, worthlessness
    hopelessness

Hypochondriacal delusions
Nihilistic delusions
Delusional misidentification

Delusions of control

Delusions of control occur when the patient explains his experiences of passivity as caused by an outside agency using machines, rays, hypnotism, magic, etc to influence him. In experiences of passivity (first rank symptoms of schizophrenia; see Table 17.5), the patient feels that his thoughts, actions or feelings are 'made' and do not originate from himself. If the phenomenon occurs in a person whose religious group believes in 'possession' by spirits, it may be difficult to distinguish from the possession state, but the latter is more akin to a transient state of depersonalization, when talking and acting in an automatic way lasts for a few hours. The fact that his religious group does not accept the phenomenon as normal distinguishes this possession state from delusions of control in which the patient believes he is made against his will to do, feel or think things.

Delusions of reference

Whereas ideas of reference are loosely held, delusions of reference are held with conviction. The person believes that incidental events, gestures or remarks (for instance, television or newspaper items) are directed at himself or refer to himself. This occurs in insecure patients with poor self-esteem arising either from a sensitive personality structure or from paranoid or affective illness (Chapter 14). It may be difficult in some cases to determine whether a patient who says he hears people talking about him is describing auditory hallucinations, which he attributes to people nearby, auditory illusions or delusions of reference.

Religious delusions

Religious delusions are most commonly seen in people with a religious upbringing or strong religious connections. Those who have been members of an evangelical church are especially likely to manifest affective or paranoid illness through religious delusions. It is sometimes necessary to interview members of the same church in order to determine whether the ideas being expressed are delusions rather than shared religious beliefs, and to know whether or not the patient has become religious since developing other signs of mental illness. These delusions often have a grandiose flavour.

Delusions of infidelity

The patient has the delusion that his sexual partner is unfaithful to him, and he behaves accordingly. This may occur as a part of various organic and functional disorders, or as an isolated delusion (see Chapter 9).

Delusions of love

These also may occur as isolated symptoms (pure erotomania, de Clerambault's syndrome) or as part of another psychiatric disorder, especially schizophrenia or manic-depressive disorder. The patient believes that some person, to whom she usually stands in a dependent position, e.g. a priest or a doctor, is in love with her in spite of his paradoxically evasive behaviour.

Grandiose delusions

Patients with grandiose delusions believe that they are special in some way. They may believe that they are of royal descent, very wealthy, geniuses, divinities, ministers, or intelligence agents.

Depressive delusions

These concern feelings of guilt, worthlessness, poverty, hopelessness and are discussed in Chapter 14.

Hypochondriacal delusions

Hypochondriasis is usually an expression of some other underlying psychiatric disorder (see Chapter 21). Hypochondriacal delusions are especially associated with depression when they concern intractable diseases, for example cancer, or have sinful implications such as venereal disease; they may arise from bodily changes such as constipation. When they occur with schizophrenia they are usually secondary to depression of mood or experience of bodily change or somatic hallucinations.

Nihilistic delusions

These involve the belief that parts of the patient or his world do not exist. For example, the patient may believe that he has no digestive tract or that a relative is dead. They occur mainly in agitated depression, but can occur in schizophrenia and organic brain disease.

Delusional misidentification

Delusional misidentification may occur as a form of delusional perception or delusional misinterpretation, as when the patient misidentifies those around him as a policemen. In the Capgras syndrome (delusion of doubles) the patient believes that people he meets (usually close relatives) have been replaced by impostors who look identical. In the Fregoli delusion, the patient believes that various people he meets are embodiments of a single person, by whom he feels persecuted. Organic brain disease should be considered in assessing patients with symptoms such as these.

CONDITIONS ASSOCIATED WITH PARANOID DELUSIONS (see Table 17.4)

The diagnosis of conditions with paranoid delusions requires a full assessment of the history and mental state, together with a physical examination, since the symptom is very non-specific. it is important to establish the development, course and duration of the symptoms; and to discover whether the premorbid personality included prominent paranoid or schizoid traits that would predispose to the development, and if drugs or alcohol are implicated. In the mental state evidence should be sought of depressive and manic syndromes and of other forms of delusions and hallucinations, particularly first rank symptoms of schizophrenia (see Table 17.5).

Paranoid states and disorders

Paranoid state, simple, is a category which appears in ICD–9 but not in DSM–III, of psychoses, acute or chronic, in which fixed and systematized delusions of influence, persecution or grandiosity are the main symptoms and in which there is no evidence of either schizophrenia or an affective psychosis. These patients would probably be diagnosed in DSM–III under the general grouping of paranoid disorder, the type being determined by details of the symptomatology.

The term paranoid disorder is used in DSM–III to classify patients with paranoid delusions who are without hallucinations or evidence of schizophrenia, major depression, mania or relevant organic disorder. The disorders are predisposed by various forms of social isolation and sensory deprivation, such as deafness. In *acute paranoid disorder*, the condition usually lasts less than six months and follows some insecurity in the patient's life, as with refugees and immigrants. Some psychogenic psychoses take this form when the diagnosis in ICD–9 would be acute paranoid reaction. *Paranoia* is a chronic paranoid disorder, usually of insidious onset. Although DSM–III restricts the diagnosis to people with delusions of a persecutory or jealous kind, many other authors would include here those with delusions of a grandiose kind and cases of erotomania and monosymptomatic delusional hypochondriasis. In ICD–9 paraphrenia is also considered under the rubric of paranoid state but this will be discussed later in the chapter. Induced psychosis or shared paranoid disorder including folie à deux has been discussed above.

Stress-induced paranoid illnesses

Stress-induced paranoid psychoses are classified in ICD–9 either as acute paranoid reaction or as psychogenic paranoid psychosis where the illness is more protracted. These diagnoses are listed under the general heading of other non-organic psychoses, which includes other pathological states related to stress; for example, those where mood disorder is the prominent feature. In DSM–III the term brief reactive psychosis is used for those illnesses which develop suddenly after a recognizable stressful event and last for between a few hours and two weeks, without any permanent residual impairment. There is emotional turmoil and perplexity, and the psychotic features may include delusions and hallucinations; hysterical dissociative phenomena may also be in

Table 17.4 Conditions associated with paranoid delusions

ICD–9	DSM–III
1 Paranoid states	*Paranoid disorders*
paranoid state, simple	acute paranoid disorder
paranoia	paranoia
induced psychosis (folie à deux)	shared paranoid disorder
paraphrenia	
2 Stress-induced	
acute paranoid reaction	brief reactive psychosis
psychogenic paranoid psychosis	
3 Schizophrenic psychosis	*Schizophrenic disorder*
paranoid	paranoid type
4 Acute schizophrenic episode	*Schizophreniform disorder*
5 Affective psychosis	*Major affective disorders*
manic illness	
depressive illness	
6 Drug, alcohol or organic psychosis	

evidence. Abnormal personalities are vulnerable to this condition, particularly those of paranoid, schizotypal or borderline types.

Paranoid schizophrenia

The criteria for the diagnosis of schizophrenia and its subtypes are shown in Tables 17.5, 17.6 and 17.7. In the paranoid type of schizophrenia the picture is dominated by persecutory delusions, grandiose delusions, delusions of jealousy, or hallucinations with a persecutory or grandiose content. A schizophreniform disorder resembles schizophrenia in its delusional and hallucinatory

Table 17.5 Schneider's first rank symptoms

1 Hearing one's thoughts spoken aloud within one's head

2 Hearing voices that comment on what one is doing at the time

3 Experiences of bodily influence

4 Thought withdrawal and other forms of thought interference

5 Thought diffusion (broadcasting)

6 Delusional perception

7 Anything in the spheres of feeling, drive and volition which is experienced as imposed on one, or influenced by others.

Table 17.6 Criteria for the diagnosis of schizophrenia: DSM-III

A At least one of the following during a phase of the illness:
  1 bizarre delusions with no possible basis in fact, e.g. delusions of control, thought alienation
  2 other delusions without persecutory or jealous content
  3 delusions with persecutory or jealous content if accompanied by hallucinations of any type
  4 auditory hallucinations: either a running commentary on the patient's behaviour or thoughts; or two or more voices conversing with each other
  5 auditory hallucinations: on a number of occasions; of more than a couple of words; unrelated to mood
  6 incoherence, marked loosening of associations, markedly illogical thinking or marked poverty of content of speech: if associated with at least one of the following:
    a blunted, flat or inappropriate affect
    b delusions or hallucinations
    c catatonic or other grossly disorganized behaviour

B Deterioration from a previous level of functioning in such areas as work, social relations and self-care

C Duration:
    The patient must have been continuously ill at some stage for six months and must be ill at present. During at least part of this six-month period there must have been symptoms from *A* (active phase), and it may or may not include a prodromal phase with clear deterioration in functioning before the active phase or a residual phase following the active phase. For diagnosis of both prodromal and residual phase at least two of the following symptoms must be present unrelated to mood or substance abuse:

    Prodromal or Residual Symptoms
    1 social isolation or withdrawal
    2 marked impairment in occupational functioning at work or home
    3 markedly abnormal behaviour
    4 marked impairment in personal hygiene and grooming
    5 blunted, flat or inappropriate affect
    6 evidence in speech of disorder of thought form
    7 bizarre ideation
    8 unusual perceptual experiences

D Full depressive or manic syndrome if present must have developed after any psychotic symptoms or last only for a relatively short period of time compared to the duration of psychotic symptoms in *A*.

E Onset of prodromal or active phase of illness before age 45

F Symptoms not due to any organic mental disorder or mental retardation

Table 17.7 Types of schizophrenia

ICD–9	DSM–III	Characteristic features
Simple type 295.0	—	Insidious onset, odd conduct, inability to meet demands of society and decline in total performance. No delusions or hallucinations
Hebephrenic type 295.1	Disorganized type 295.1x	Frequent incoherence, no systematized delusions; blunted, inappropriate, silly affect
Catatonic type 295.2	Catatonic type 295.2x	Catatonic symptoms
Paranoid type 295.3	Paranoid type 295.3x	Delusions/hallucinations with persecutory or grandiose content; delusions of jealousy
—	Schizophreniform disorder 295.40	Short duration: two weeks to six months
Acute schizophrenic episode 295.4	—	Dream-like state with slight clouding of consciousness and perplexity; often relatively short duration
Latent schizophrenia 295.5	—	Eccentric or inconsequential behaviour; anomalies of affect giving the impression of schizophrenia without any definite schizophrenic symptoms
Residual schizophrenia 295.6	Residual type 295.6x	Continuing evidence of illness, blunted affect, withdrawal, odd behaviour, formal thought disorder, previous episode with prominent symptoms but no psychotic symptoms needing action at present
Schizoaffective type 295.7	Schizoaffective disorder 295.70	Symptoms of both affective and schizophrenic illness; cannot be diagnosed as one of the two
Other 295.8	—	Schizophrenia of specified type not classifiable under 295.0–295.7
—	Undifferentiated type 295.9x	Permanent delusions, hallucinations, incoherence or grossly disorganized behaviour not fitting other types of schizophrenia
Unspecified 295.9	—	To be used only as a last resort

symptoms but is of limited duration (more than two weeks or less than six months including any prodromal phase). The personality is then restored without a residual schizophrenia defect. In the ICD–9, the most appropriate classification would probably be acute schizophrenia episode (295.4).

Paraphrenia is the diagnostic term given to illnesses which resemble paranoid schizophrenia without thought disorder, blunting of affect or deterioration in personality. Hallucinations, often in several modalities, are particularly common. In clinical practice this term is often used where the onset is late and where the delusional system and hallucinations remain comparatively circumscribed and do not invade other aspects of the patient's personality. Thus the patient may have delusions of persecution by neighbours by which he is not troubled when on holiday. This syndrome is classified under paranoid states in ICD–9 but is not recognized as a distinct entity in DSM–III.

Affective illnesses

The occurrence of paranoid delusions in depressive illness and mania have been discussed in Chapters 14 and 16.

Organic disorders associated with paranoid delusions

In an organic delusional syndrome, delusions occur without clouding of consciousness, intellectual impairment, or hallucinations, and there is evidence of a specific organic aetiological factor, (see Table 17.8). If hallucinations are more rank symptoms (see Table 17.5). According to described as an organic hallucinosis (e.g. alcoholic hallucinosis). Organic confusional states (delirium

Table 17.8 Organic causes of delusional syndromes

Drugs:	
Psychostimulants	Amphetamine methylphenidate pemoline cocaine
Psychotomimetics	phencyclidine cannabis
Appetite suppressants	diethylpropion
Alcohol	
Dopamine agonists	(bromocriptine etc., L-dopa)
Corticosteroids	
Metabolic disorders	myxoedema
Organic brain disease	temporal lobe epilepsy neurosyphilis Huntington's chorea dementia

and dementia) may lead to the development of delusions. In delirium, the delusions arise through misinterpretation, illusions and hallucinatory experiences. In dementia, paranoid ideation may arise in response to forgetfulness or to other psychological deficits or to the changing attitudes of others around them. However, there is a particular tendency for paranoid delusions to occur in pre-senile dementia of Pick's type and in Huntington's chorea.

The psychotic symptoms produced by these organic illnesses and drugs may include the first rank symptoms (see Table 17.5). According to Schneider the presence of a symptom of the first rank is diagnostic of schizophrenia only if it occurs in clear consciousness and in the absence of coarse brain disease, although the extent to which these symptoms are highly suggestive of schizophrenia rather than pathognomonic is currently under debate. A psychosis closely similar to paranoid schizophrenia may be produced by amphetamine-like drugs, dopamine agonists and cannabis. The subject may experience first rank symptoms such as thought alienation and experiences of passivity, but being aware of having taken a drug, will not necessarily have secondary delusional ideas of influence from an outside agency. Concurrent drug abuse should be suspected in every young person who develops paranoid delusions, or when an in-patient's psychotic disorder worsens unexpectedly after a period of leave during which he may have had access to drugs.

PSYCHOSIS AND MENTAL HANDICAP

Patients whose communication is limited by low intellectual capacity may present with strange ideas and odd behaviour. This is a potential diagnostic pitfall and when seeking to establish the presence of schizophrenia and other paranoid psychoses, attention must be paid to the patient's intellectual level and general mode of functioning and ways of reacting to stress. However, the converse is also true, namely that it is important not to attribute abnormalities in the mental state of mentally handicapped patients solely to their mental handicap without considering other possibilities.

CASE HISTORY

LAVINIA ENTWHISTLE

Mrs Lavinia Entwhistle was a 58-year-old divorcee who had emigrated to Spain some five years previously. She was referred by her son and daughter-in-law whom she was visiting in England. They were worried by her insistence that a wealthy financier — Mr X — was interested in marrying her. Further enquiries had shown that this financier was in fact already happily married. When confronted with this Mrs Entwhistle said she was convinced he would leave his wife. When asked how she had first met this man she said that they had never actually met but his actions showed that he loved her. One action was to buy a villa in close proximity to hers; another was to go to that villa for a fortnight's holiday at the time of her birthday. It was suggested to her that she might be mistaken but at this she became very angry and accused her children of being against her and trying to deprive her of the chance of happiness. They tried to persuade her to see a psychiatrist but not surprisingly she refused and promptly left their house and returned to Spain, vowing never to see or even speak to them again.

In the following months she began to run up large hotel bills when she would go away for weeks on end to luxury hotels; when it was time to pay she would say that Mr X would settle the bill. For the same reason she stopped paying her mortgage on her villa and got into debt at the local shops. Finally, summonses were taken out against her not only by the shopkeepers and institutions to whom she was in debt but also by Mr X.

Her reaction to this was to maintain that she was being persecuted by people who were jealous of Mr X's interest in her. She refused to accept that Mr X had taken legal action against her, and insisted that this was part of the same conspiracy. At this point her son was asked to come over to Spain to try and sort the situation out. Though Mrs Entwhistle once again refused to see a psychiatrist, she was told by the courts that unless she did so she was at risk of being sent to prison or deported from Spain. She reluctantly agreed to come back to England for a psychiatric interview, 'to show them she was sane'.

At interview it transpired that Mrs Entwhistle was the youngest by some years of three sisters born to a wealthy Yorkshire wool merchant who had lost his money during the depression, when Mrs Entwhistle was seven years old. By this time her sisters, who were thirteen and fifteen years older than she was, had already left home and made good marriages. The remaining family, Mr and Mrs Entwhistle and Lavinia, had to leave their large detached house to go into a small rented terraced house, and Lavinia had to leave her private school to join the rough and tumble of the local state school. This proved quite a shock for her and she found it very difficult to settle in. The other children teased her for being posh and putting on airs and graces but this only led to her becoming more aloof and isolated. At times she retreated into a fantasy would of her own where she was a princess in a golden palace with all the trinkets that money could buy. At home she was the only child — her sisters rarely visited, her father had started drinking and her parents rowed frequently, eventually to be divorced when Lavinia was twenty-two.

After leaving school Lavinia went to secretarial college and got a job as a secretary in a local business. There she proved herself to be efficient and soon rose to be personal assistant to the managing director. She had no friends either inside or outside work, tending to put people off with her aloof and haughty manner. However, the managing director was also fairly isolated; the two of them became increasingly friendly and married just before her thirtieth birthday. Their one and only child — a boy — was born one year later. At first the marriage was a happy one with the couple being self-sufficient but after eight years her husband started to make excuses for not coming home for dinner and for working late at the office. Initially Mrs Entwhistle not only believed her husband but took pity on him for having to work such long hours. But gossip spread around the town that he was having an affair with his new personal assistant, a young, attractive and vivacious girl. Mrs Entwhistle dismissed all this as mere rumour spread by those who were jealous of her happiness and success. However, one day when putting her husband's clothes away she discovered a bunch of love-letters written by this girl. There then followed a bitter and acrimonious divorce during which her husband said that the reason he had had an affair was that she had no fun in her, was always suspicious of others and would never make friends.

Following the divorce, Mrs Entwhistle wrapped herself up in caring for her eight-year-old son. She was overprotective towards him and very careful about who he mixed with — no one was ever good enough for him. As her son grew up it became apparent that he was very athletic and good at sports and this provided him with an entry into the school social set-up. This weakened the ties between mother and son and as she had made no friends she became increasingly isolated and bitter. At the age of twenty her son met a vivacious, attractive girl, whom the mother identified with the personal assistant who had stolen her husband. Try as the young couple might, Mrs Entwhistle never warmed towards her future daughter-in-law, refusing to go to the wedding or, initially, to visit the young couple. Later when she did go round to the house she virtually ignored her daughter-in-law.

Finally three years ago, after they had been married for two years, she emigrated to Spain. She remained isolated and made no friends in Spain, spending every evening on her own. Some of the other expatriates made overtures towards her but they were always rejected as 'only being out to get something from her'.

There was no past or family psychiatric history except for her father's drinking, and she had been a teetotaller all her life.

The mental state examination revealed a rather hostile but sad-looking woman who admitted she was unhappy but had no impairment of sleep or appetite and no suicidal thoughts. She was guarded in her replies to questioning about her time in Spain and in particular her relationship with Mr X. However, it transpired that though she had never talked to Mr X she was absolutely convinced he loved her and wanted to marry her. She was unshakeable on this. She also insisted that other people were jealous of this relationship and would take any steps to prevent it, including spying on her and bugging her telephone. She said that she was sure Mr X had paid all the outstanding bills and the shopkeepers and others were lying to get at her and to demean her in Mr X's eyes. There were no ideas of influence, no hallucinations and her cognitive state was intact.

Questions

What is the diagnosis?
Why have these symptoms arisen in this woman at this time?
Can any predictions be made about the son's future?

Though delusions of love may occur on their own (de Clerambault's syndrome), in this case they are associated with paranoid delusions and the differential diagnosis is of conditions in which paranoid delusions occur. This lady clearly had a paranoid/schizoid personality upon which have been superimposed the delusional ideas. There is no evidence of schizophrenic first rank symptoms, and though she is depressed there is nothing else to suggest a major depressive disorder, nor is there any evidence of alcohol or drug abuse. It would be wise to rule out organic causes of paranoid illness, e.g. endocrine disorders. The most likely diagnosis is either a simple paranoid state: 297.0 ICD–9; this diagnosis does not feature in DSM–III, or a paranoid disorder: paranoia 297.10 (DSM III) or 297.1 (ICD–9).

Mrs Entwhistle's paranoid/schizoid personality makes her particularly prone to social isolation and thus to developing a paranoid state/disorder consequent on this. Her paranoid/schizoid personality would be related to her traumatic experiences as the 'only' child of a family who had fallen on hard times with parents who quarrelled. There were already signs in childhood of difficulty in making relationships and of escape into a fantasy life. Her parents' marital problems would predispose her to vulnerability in this area and it is not surprising that her marriage broke down, nor that she developed delusions of love for someone who would perhaps have been not too dissimilar to her father before his business failed.

Symptoms have probably arisen now because her son's marriage has taken away the only real relationship she ever made and since going to Spain she has become even more isolated.

His parents' divorce and his mother's overprotectiveness and suspiciousness would suggest that her son's area of vulnerability would be in the spheres of social and sexual relationships. However, his athletic prowess at school with his resulting popularity appears to have counteracted his mother's influence. The same is true of his marriage to a warm, vivacious girl who appears to be the opposite of his mother. It is possible that if his marriage ended in circumstances in which he saw himself as inadequate — e.g., his wife has an affair which she flaunted in his face — he might become paranoid like his mother, though his social abilities would militate against this.

18

Voices, visions and other perceptual abnormalities

The conscious awareness of incoming sensations is the result of a complex sequence involving sensory organs, neurological pathways and higher cerebral functions. Sensations are attended to selectively, depending on their importance and emotional connotations. Perceptions are learnt and interpreted by higher centres as studies of patients with agnosias demonstrates; in visual agnosias, for example, although the visual apparatus is normal, patients cannot identify objects despite being able to see and copy them. It is not surprising, therefore, that perceptual abnormalities are common in people with organic and functional psychiatric disorders.

SENSORY DISTORTIONS

Perceptual abnormalities can be divided into distortions and deceptions (Table 18.1). Sensory distortion occurs when some features of the percept are changed in form, quality or intensity. Many distortions are the result of neurological disease, especially of the special senses.

Changes in form occur visually as micropsia or macropsia: objects appearing smaller or larger than they are. Both micropsia and macropsia occur in the presence of retinal damage, may indicate damage to the visual association areas in the temporal lobe when associated with temporal lobe (complex partial) epilepsy, and may occur in migraine.

Qualitative changes can be induced by psychoactive drugs of which lysergic acid diethylamide, (LSD) is a prime example. LSD commonly induces changes in the colour, texture and significance of visual perceptions. Changes in intensity can also be produced by drugs, so that sights and sounds appear brighter and louder or may be diminished. Increase in intensity (hyperacusis) is a classic symptom in post-traumatic neurosis following head injury, and also occurs in anxiety states. Depressed patients may be aware of hypoacusis (decreased intensity); one depressed patient, for example, said, 'Depression takes at least 50 watts off an 150-watt light bulb'.

SENSORY DECEPTIONS

Illusions

Illusions are false perceptions of external sensory stimuli. They occur in conditions where sensations are not clear, for example, visually at night, or auditorily against a noisy background, or where attention is reduced, for example in acute confusional states. Illusions are also associated with the affective state and are most likely to occur when people are apprehensive or afraid; for example, when walking alone on a dark night, misidentifying a tree as a man waiting to attack.

Illusions must be distinguished from intellectual misinterpretations, where individuals do not

Table 18.1 Abnormal percept

Distortion		Deception
Changes in:		
form	micropsia	illusions
	macropsia	pseudohallucinations
		hallucinations
quality		
intensity	hypoacusis	
	hyperacusis	

understand what they are perceiving; for example believing that one heard a car backfire when in fact one heard the sound of gunshot.

Hallucinations

Hallucinations, which occur in all sensory modalities, are experienced as true percepts but arise in the absence of external sensory stimuli. They are not perceived in the mind, and so are not images, but in the external environment or the body of the hallucinating person. Hallucinations may be *elementary*, such as single sounds, or flashes of light; or *complex* and fully formed such as voices or animals. The person must experience the percept as real before an hallucination can be diagnosed, and although some chronically hallucinated patients may *learn* that these percepts are unreal, they are still hallucinating because they continue to be *experienced* as true. On occasion, it may be difficult to distinguish delusional belief from hallucinatory experience, particularly in patients who cannot express themselves easily. Hallucinations are frequently explained delusionally: 'The voices I hear talking behind me are the television camera crew who are filming me all the time'. The discrimination between 'I know people are talking about me' and 'I hear people talking about me' is not always easy to establish. Confusion sometimes exists between hallucinations and delusional perceptions or misinterpretations (Chapter 17). In the latter the percept is real but it is interpreted delusionally.

Functional hallucinations are false perceptions which arise at the same time as a true one. Some patients hallucinate on each occasion that the associated stimulus is experienced.

Pseudohallucinations

There is more than one definition of pseudohallucination, which limits its use as a concept. It remains, however, somewhat of a minefield in postgraduate examination vivas, and some familiarity with the term is recommended.

The most widely accepted definition is: a false perception which occurs outside the mind (in objective space) but which is recognized at the time as being unreal since it either lacks some qualities of a real percept, or has some additional qualities which make it appear unreal — an 'as if' experience. Some religious revelations fall into this category; for example, a vision of the Virgin Mary appearing in two dimensions as if a picture were projected into space.

Pseudohallucinations are said to occur if the subject recognizes the unreality of a perception in retrospect. Since it is difficult to know how much time should elapse before an interpretation is 'retrospective' this definition does not usefully aid discrimination between pseudo- and true hallucinations.

A further definition is that pseudohallucinations are excessively vivid mental images perceived in subjective as opposed to objective space, and are never experienced as real. Mental imagery is the term given to experiences with have some qualities of percepts but which are 'seen in the mind's eye' and are never attributed to external sensory stimuli.

Distinction between pseudohallucinations and true hallucinations

If abnormal perceptual experiences are envisaged along a continuum with mental images at one end, true hallucinations at the other, and pseudohallucinations in the centre, it can be understood that different definitions arise depending on different cut-off points along the continuum. In clinical practice the distinction between imagery and pseudohallucinations is much less important than that between pseudo- and true hallucinations. The appearance of reality and the occurrence outside the self are the two aspects of true hallucination which should be established before the percept is so defined.

The situation is further complicated by the fact that certain abnormal phenomena are classed as pseudohallucinations by some authorities and as true hallucinations by others. The false perceptions which occur in bereavement, such as seeing or hearing the dead loved one, fall into this category, as does the 'phantom limb' experience of amputees. Autoscopy or *doppelgänger*, the experience of seeing oneself outside one's body, is similarly classified as either experience.

In clinical practice, therefore, each abnormal

perception should be classified on the basis of the patient's individual experience, and a verbatim account should be made so that the evidence for a classification is apparent.

MODALITIES

Visual hallucinations

Elementary hallucinations of flashing lights or colours may occur. Complex hallucinations are usually of living things such as people's faces, or animals, but may be of inanimate objects. Visual hallucinations may occur in addition to, or instead of, normal visual perceptions.

Auditory hallucinations

People's voices are the most common complex auditory hallucination, although music, either continuously or in snatches, also occurs. Hallucinatory voices may be those of people recognized by the patient, or of strangers, may be of either sex, and may be quite distinct. Alternatively, they may be mumbling and impossible to identify. Voices may be perceived as single or coming from many different people, and they may address the person or talk to each other, referring to the subject. They may be intermittent or continuous. They may be derogatory and critical, or cheerful and expansive. They are usually experienced outside the body, at head height or above, but may be heard as coming from the body. Voices which are heard (as opposed to felt) inside the head are true hallucinations if they are perceived as real. Auditory hallucinations may appear to arise from particular places or objects — for example, a particular doorway, or the television — or to come from any direction. The details of auditory hallucinations must be established since they are of diagnostic significance (see below).

Olfactory and gustatory hallucinations

Hallucinations in these modalities are usually of pungent, unpleasant smells and tastes. They may be recognized as familiar by the patient: for example, bad food or noxious gases; or may be a completely new experience which is difficult for the patient to describe in words. Sometimes complaints of abnormal smells and taste are delusional rather than hallucinatory; for example when the patient complains that his food is bad because he knows someone is poisoning it rather than because its taste is different.

Tactile hallucinations

False perceptions of the sence of touch can occur either superficially, affecting the skin, or deeply, inside the body. Superficial tactile hallucinations are commonly sensations of crawling, scratching, or change in temperature. Deeply seated hallucinations may be of pain in viscera or feelings of manipulation inside joints. Sexual hallucinations occur, where women experience interference in the vagina.

THE PATTERN OF HALLUCINATIONS IN PSYCHIATRIC ILLNESS

Certain hallucinations are strong diagnostic indicators of particular psychiatric illnesses and it is the identification of these illnesses which makes the precise nature of hallucinations so important to establish.

Organic conditions

Acute or chronic brain disease or dysfunction can produce hallucinations of any type, but the most important diagnostic association is with visual hallucinations. True visual hallucinations must be presumed organic in origin until proved otherwise.

Acute organic psychoses

Delirium results in a multiplicity of abnormal perceptions of which illusions are the most common. Patients frequently misperceive people such as nurses or family as threatening persecutors or jailers. In addition, visual hallucinations occur, characteristically of small animals which are usually frightening. On occasion the hallucination is appealing, as with the patient who was found under his bed trying to encourage the little badger who had just run under it to come out and join him. Lilliputian hallucinations are described where tiny animals and people are seen enacting scenes in front of the patient. Visual hallucinations are multiple but short-lived in acute organic states. Fragments of speech and elementary auditory hallucinations occur as do superficial tactile hallucinations.

Drug-induced organic states may be associated with particular abnormal percepts. For example, LSD and phencyclidine produce fantastic and bizarre visual hallucinations in addition to sensory distortions. Cocaine intoxication is associated with formication: a sensation as of insects crawling under the skin.

Chronic organic states

Patients with dementia may hallucinate but in advanced cases may not be able clearly to describe their experiences. Visual and/or auditory hallucinations may be inferred by the patient's behaviour: for example, the holding of an animated, if incoherent, conversation with someone evidently in the room with him.

Focal lesions

Lesions in the occipital cortex or cortical association areas can produce elementary visual hallucinations such as flashes of light, or complex experiences which are usually stereotyped. Visual hallucinations are more likely to occur in blind areas of the visual field. Migraine produces characteristic percepts: blind spots and series of inter-related shimmering lines, so-called fortification spectra.

Partial epilepsies are associated with hallucinations at the beginning of the attack — the aura. These can be of localizing significance, for example, olfactory and gustatory hallucinations in epilepsies with a temporal lobe focus. Posterior temporal foci produce visual and auditory auras which in some cases are combined: for example a visual hallucination of a person who speaks.

Patients with parietal lobe damage may perceive part of their body as not belonging to them, and hence complain about the other person who lies in bed with them. This is not hallucinatory but an illusion, since the abnormal percept occurs in the presence of a sensory stimulus.

Disorders of sense organs

Local disease of special sensory organs can produce hallucinations, usually of an elementary nature: for example, the tinnitus of inner ear disease, and the sensation of falling flashes of light in those who are blind. Sometimes these percepts are very distressing and their emotional content reflects the psychopathology of the patient; for example, an elderly man, recently blinded by glaucoma, experienced frequent hallucinations of sexually provocative but dangerous and predatory women.

Functional psychoses

Schizophrenia

Auditory hallucinations are the abnormal percepts most characteristic of schizophrenia. Certain types of auditory hallucination are considered of significance, in the absence of brain disease, for a diagnosis of schizophrenia. There are some differences in detail between different systems (Table 18.2) but there is broad agreement. Hearing one's own thoughts spoken aloud, either as they are thought or immediately afterwards; hearing voices speaking to each other about one, or hearing one or more voice continuously commenting on one's actions are characteristic. Voices in the second person,

Table 18.2 Hallucinations of diagnostic significance in schizophrenia — in the absence of brain disease

Schneider's 1st rank symptoms
Hearing one's own thoughts spoken aloud

Continuous third person voices discussing one, or giving a running commentary

Somatic hallucinations when part of passivity — 'made' experiences

DSM III
One voice with a running commentary on the individual's thought or actions

Two or more voices conversing together

Occurring on several occasions: more than one or two words, not related to mood

Of any type *if* associated with delusions of persecution or jealousy.

that is addressing the patient directly with comments or commands, occur commonly, as do elementary auditory percepts; these, however, are not diagnostic of the condition.

Experiences in other modalities are not infrequent, but not useful for diagnosis, except in the case of somatic hallucinations occurring as part of a passivity phenomenon. Bizarre tactile hallucinations, especially of deep sensations, occur, as do olfactory and gustatory perceptions usually associated with delusions of being gassed or poisoned. Visual hallucinations do occur but are less prominent than auditory ones. Care must be taken to elicit the abnormalities with accuracy; for example, a patient who said that doves flew past him when he was standing by the open window of the ward was thought to be describing visual hallucinations. Closer questioning revealed that he felt birds' feet land on his shoulder and heard wings flapping past him; although he saw nothing abnormal he knew that these were white doves.

Delusions of parasitism (Ekbom's syndrome) may be a monosymptomatic delusional psychosis or a variant of paraphrenia where the patient believes his person and his surroundings are infested by insects. Tactile hallucinations of crawling or irritation occur in this condition.

The emotional significance of hallucinations in schizophrenia is variable. Acutely ill patients are frightened and angered by the alien presences which are constantly talking, but when these persist chronically, many patients become unconcerned and apathetic about them. On occasions, schizophrenic patients derive some kind of comfort in their isolation from their accompanying voices and miss them if they disappear.

Manic depressive psychoses

Mania Auditory hallucinations occur uncommonly in severe mania. They are transient and not continuous and are characteristically of voices talking to the patient in an expansive manner with a grandiose content; saying for example, 'You are very rich'. True hallucinations in other modalities are not symptoms of mania.

Depression Severe depressive psychosis is associated with auditory hallucinations in the second person. These are intermittent and their content is depressive and condemnatory. 'You deserve to die, kill yourself' is a typical example. Suicidal attempts are occasionally preceded by hallucinations of this type.

Alcoholic hallucinosis

Alcoholic hallucinosis takes the form of vivid, continuous auditory hallucinations which are threatening or insulting. It is distinguished from organic brain syndromes associated with alcohol dependence by the fact that it occurs in clear consciousness. Its aetiology is unclear, however, and the natural history of the condition is varied; some patients go on to develop a frank paranoid psychosis, whilst in others evidence of dementia becomes apparent with time.

Neurotic disorders

Most perceptual abnormalities described by neurotic patients are not true hallucinations, but are either imagery, illusions or pseudohallucinations. However, visual hallucinations have been described in hysteria, and some patients with anxiety, fatigue, social isolation or combinations of these may experience transient hallucinations to a greater extent than those abnormal percepts which occur, occasionally, in people without psychiatric disease.

HALLUCINATIONS OCCURRING IN NORMAL PEOPLE

Transient hallucinations, especially at times of fatigue, can occur in the absence of psychiatric disease. Most commonly these are elementary auditory hallucinations of one or two words heard indistinctly. When the latter occur in the transition from wakefulness to sleep, they are called hypnagogic, and if when waking from sleep, they are hypnopompic. Hypnagogic and hypnopompic hallucinations also occur in narcolepsy (see Chapter 5).

Autoscopic (doppelgänger) hallucinations also occur in normal people, while recently bereaved people, in the searching and the pining stages of grief, commonly experience the voice of the loved one calling their name, or the sight of them standing near them in the house, for example. As mentioned earlier, these are sometimes classed as pseudohallucinations and sometimes as true ones, and the distinction is made on whether the person experiences these percepts as real or not. Some of these experiences are illusions, as when a person misperceives someone walking towards them in the street as the lost loved one; but whatever phenomenon is described, it is important that the bereaved person is reassured of its normal origin.

CASE HISTORY

JOSEPHINE WARNER

Josephine Warner, a 35-year-old woman was brought to Casualty one evening by her second husband. She had been agitated and acting strangely for about a week, and earlier that evening had repeatedly gone to an upstairs flat to ask whether they had children, crying, there. She had been bewildered at finding no children present, and had only been temporarily reassured, insisting on going upstairs again a few minutes later to check. Mr Warner said that for several days she had been withdrawn and preoccupied and would often stop what she was doing to go to the window to look out; seemed, from time to time to be listening to something, and over the last forty-eight hours had several times asked him if he could hear a voice. She had been unable to go to her work as a bank clerk for four days, and had been sleeping poorly. For several days she had been reluctant to leave their flat.

Mrs Warner was unable to add much to this history; her concentration was poor; she was preoccupied and perplexed, and seemed to have difficulty in marshalling her thoughts. Her speech and actions were slow, and the interview was punctuated by her asking if the doctor heard the noise of children outside — invariably following some sound from outside the interview room. She said that she had been hearing children crying and calling for their mother, and had also heard different voices speaking to her, saying things like, 'Why don't you phone John?' (her first

husband). She was unable to distinguish any other content. She had been reluctant to go out because people seemed to be talking about her in the street, and she was worried by the television which appeared to be broadcasting information about her in some way.

She appeared depressed in mood, could not say how she felt about the future, and sat, dejectedly, with tears streaming down her face. She knew she was unwell, although she denied having felt like this before; she also said that she thought her ex-husband was, in some way, organizing things to make her ill. On direct questioning, the only other abnormality was that she said she thought that she smelt; and was sure that the reason she had been asked that was because the doctor could smell her odour. This was very distressing to her, since she was normally a fastidious person.

Her husband gave further details of Mrs Warner's past history. Her early life had no particularly unusual features, and the only history of psychiatric illness in the family was in her elder sister who had had two admissions to hospital for psychiatric treatment; each admission had lasted about 3 months and she had completely recovered from each illness. Mrs Warner's first marriage, at the age of twenty-one, had lasted eight years. She had a disastrous obstetric history, with three miscarriages before she gave birth to a son, who died after forty-eight hours. She had developed a puerperal psychosis a week after her son's birth, and had a further episode of mental illness 4 years later, six months after her divorce. She had been well for the previous five years, and had been happily married for the last three. Six weeks before, her nine-year-old nephew, of whom she was very fond, had been killed in a road traffic accident.

Questions

What is the diagnostic significance of Mrs Warner's perceptual abnormalities?
What is the differential diagnosis?
What is the role of stress in the aetiology?
Mrs Warner is suffering from more than one kind of auditory perceptual abnormality. Her experiences of hearing crying children are hallucinatory

— there is no evidence that such sounds are audible to anyone else, and she describes a clear example of a voice talking to her in the second person. Her perception during the interview of the sounds of children may have been hallucinatory, but apparently occurred in response to some other sound — this experience may have been an auditory illusion, a functional hallucination (a rare hallucination regularly occuring at the same time as a normal perception) or a misinterpretation of the significance of ordinary perceptions. At this stage in the assessment it is impossible to differentiate these phenomena with greater clarity.

Similarly, the nature of her ideas of reference is difficult to elucidate. She may be experiencing clear perceptions in the absence of auditory sensory input when in the street, or she may be misperceiving snatches of ordinary conversation which she misinterprets as referring to her. Whether her ideas of reference are held with delusional intensity has not been tested so far in the mental state examination. Neither is it clear whether her statement about smelling bad is based on an olfactory hallucination, or a delusion, or both.

Diagnostically, these experiences point to an affective illness. Her auditory hallucinations are in the second person, and in the context of her past and recent experiences of childhood death, are depressive in content. An abnormal belief about smelling bad is most often depressive, although if this is founded on an abnormal olfactory perception, an affective cause is unlikely.

The differential diagnosis is between depressive psychosis, psychogenic paranoid psychosis and paranoid state. There is no evidence of alcohol abuse, which excludes a diagnosis of alcoholic hallucinosis. The evidence in favour of a depressive psychosis is, in addition to the hallucinations, the fact that she is depressed in mood with psychomotor retardation. She also has a past personal and family history of severe episodic mental illness which apparently remits completely between attacks. Her sleep is disturbed, although the details of this are unclear. Although her ideas of reference about people in the street and programmes on the television are compatible with a diagnosis of depression, they are equally so with that of paranoid psychosis, and so are not of diagnostic significance in this case.

However, she is beginning to develop a paranoid delusional system which centres around her first husband acting maliciously towards her. She feels distressed and angry, but does not feel that this treatment is deserved; she is not expressing feelings of guilt. A diagnosis of paranoid state or disorder is unlikely since she has both hallucinations and evidence of a depressive disorder. A stress-induced paranoid illness is a strong possibility and its exact classification into a psychogenic paranoid psychosis, and acute paranoid reaction (ICD–9) or a brief reactive psychosis (DSM–III) would depend on its duration. This diagnosis is supported by the fact that all her episodes of illness have centred around an area of major stress in her life. However, although earlier episodes have developed quickly following the stress, there has been a delay of several weeks on this occasion. It is important to establish how, and how quickly, her previous illnesses responded to treatment, before this diagnosis is discarded.

At this early stage of assessment, then, the diagnosis lies between depressive illness and stress-induced paranoid disorder. Further observation of her mental state, particularly her paranoid beliefs and her depressive signs and symptoms, will be required. Whatever the final diagnosis, there seems little doubt that the stress involved with her own failure as a mother has been important in the past and the loss of a favourite nephew — who was about the same age as her own son would have been had he lived — is likely to be implicated now. It may not be a causal relationship, but certainly appears to be determining the content of her mental state, which is largely concerned with children in distress and danger.

19

Disorders of memory, orientation and concentration — 'confusion'

The single term, memory, covers the complex functions of processing incoming information from sensory perception. Different perceptions are dealt with in different ways at different times, both within and between individuals, and some information is remembered for years whilst some is barely registered, or forgotten almost immediately.

Memory can be divided into four functions: registration, retention, recognition and recall. *Registration* is the first step, in that it is the degree to which a percept is attended to and the selection of items to be remembered. *Retention* is the storage function, and *recognition* refers to the process whereby an item in the memory store is perceived as relevant to the matter in hand. *Recall* is the retrieval of a memory to conscious awareness. It is clear that not all perceptions are processed through all these stages, and that memory is selective. Evidence from experimental psychology suggests that memory storage is a three-stage process of different levels or 'boxes' (Figure 3).

SENSORY STORES

Unprocessed information is held at peripheral sites of sensory input for a very short time — less than one second. These sites provide continuity of perception and presumably allow time for information to be processed.

SHORT TERM MEMORY

This store has a limited capacity and items of information are held for a period of about 30 seconds before they are either lost or stored for a longer time. Rehearsal (repetition) of items increases the time of retention. An example is the effect of rehearsal on the memory of a name of someone to whom one has just been introduced.

LONG TERM MEMORY

Permanent memory of certain items of information is stored long term. Memories held in this

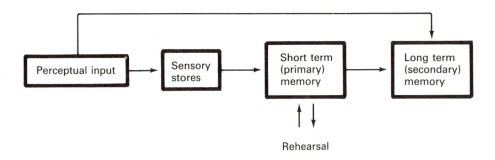

Figure 3

large-capacity store are reorganized and associated with other memories in individual ways by different people. There are at least two components potentially of clinical significance in this store: firstly, the memory of language and general knowledge which is common to many; and secondly, specific individual experiences of events.

It is important to note that clinicians in describing disorders of memory often use 'short term' and 'long term' in less precise ways. Short term memory is often taken to mean recent memory, i.e. memories of several minutes or hours and long term to memories of events of several weeks, months or years ago.

ANATOMY AND PHYSIOLOGY OF MEMORY

The hippocampus and the temporal lobes are the sites of the cerebral cortex most important for memory function, although more precise location has yet to be determined. Studies of brain-damaged individuals indicate that the left and right hemispheres are the sites for short term stores of verbal and visual information respectively. The physiology of memory is similarly poorly understood, but it is likely that sensory and short term storage is in the form of electrical impulses and that long term memory is mediated by chemical changes either in neurotransmitters or possibly in RNA.

NORMAL VARIATIONS IN MEMORY

There is a wide variation in individual memory capabilities, and many people are proud of a 'good' memory or complain of a constitutionally poor one. Some people seem to have an infinite ability to remember minutiae for a long period of time and retrieve them quickly and accurately, whilst others retain the common ability of children to remember visual perceptions absolutely by re-perceiving them in the mind's eye (photographic memory, or eidetic imagery).

Higher intelligence and good memory are to some extent related but education is an important factor. Much of the teaching in primary and secondary school is devoted to improving learning, and people with good memory usually have particular techniques of rehearsal and a well developed ability to remember information by associating items in terms of meaning, sound or imagery.

MEMORY PROBLEMS

Difficulties in memory are rarely presented to doctors in isolation but may be associated with other symptoms, or admitted to on direct questioning. Patients may have no complaints at all about their memory but deficits become obvious in the mental state examination or are complained of by those with whom the patient lives. The complaint of poor memory is fairly meaningless unless further specified. It may involve any one or more of the processes described above or in fact be unrelated to memory at all: for example, a patient may complain of memory failure when he is too embarrassed to admit that he cannot read. It is essential, therefore, before formal memory testing is embarked upon, to establish exactly what the patient means, with examples of his memory failure, the circumstances under which it occurs and so on. Many people associate poor memory with going mad and in some circumstances it may be preferable to acknowledge the symptom but postpone extensive testing to a later interview when the patient is less anxious.

MEMORY TESTING

The initial task is to identify which functions may be affected: registration, retention, recognition or recall; and whether the patient is complaining of a global loss or decrease of memory, or of a failure of specific memories. More detailed clinical testing should then take place, and the patient may subsequently be referred for psychometric assessment.

Clinical test

Orientation for time, place and person should be tested (see below), and the level of consciousness should be known. Detailed assessment of memory is at best unreliable and at worst impossible, unless the patient's consciousness is clear and his concentration adequate. Memory for past and recent personal events and general knowledge should be tested separately (see Table 19.1); although there are several recommended short schedules which can be used as a screen and include simple orientation, memory for names and addresses, and a few general knowledge questions. Whatever means of testing are employed, answers must be recorded verbatim, both to establish a base line level of functioning, and to ensure that answers are only not recorded as right or wrong, but that evidence suggestive of perseveration, guessing or concrete thinking is not missed.

In addition to these questions, new learning ability should be tested. It is assumed that the doctor will have introduced him/herself as a matter of course; is this name remembered later in the interview? If not, it should be repeated, the patient should be asked to repeat it back immediately, and if it is correct, he should be asked to remember it for a few minutes when it should be asked again. A name and address should be tested in the same way. It is essential that immediate memory is tested separately from recall after several minutes; if this is omitted, failure of concentration or short term memory will be missed and the fault wrongly attributed to a failure of recognition and/or recall. Verbal memory can also be tested by use one of the Babcock sentences: 'One thing a nation must have to be rich and great is a large secure supply of wood': or the two sentence test: 'The river passes by with a soft murmuring sound. The cricket match was won in the very last over'. Non-impaired patients of normal intelligence should be

Table 19.1 Mental state assessment of cognitive state

Testing for past personal events

    Year of birth
    Place of birth
    Name of school
    Age at first employment
    Type of first employment
    Age at and year of marriage
    Date of death of parents
    Years of birth and names of children

Other questions such as: number of jobs, house moves, year of death of spouse, retirement, number of hospitalizations etc., may be relevant depending on the patient's history

Recent personal events

    Date of hospital admission or visit to outpatient department
    Names of family members accompanying patient
    Names and functions of people seen today
    What was eaten for breakfast/lunch
    What was on today's television, in newspapers

Other questions: memory for significant recent personal event, for example accident, bereavement if appropriate to history

General events

    Item of recent news
    Name of monarch and other members of Royal Family
    Name of Prime Minister and party in power
    Previous Prime Minister
    Date of start and end of both World Wars

Other questions depend on age, interests and educational level of patient, for example: sporting events, leading football teams etc., industrial and political events, popular songs and shows able to repeat these without error. Finally, memory for numbers should be assessed by asking the patient to repeat a series of unrelated numbers forwards and backwards. Most people can repeat seven forwards and five backwards.

Other cerebral functions

If significant errors occur in the above tests, other cerebral functions should be assessed. Visuospatial difficulties are tested by asking the patient to judge distances between objects around him and to draw and copy simple figures such as a cube and clock face. Dressing apraxia and other failures to perform purposeful movements should be assessed, as should right/left orientation, co-ordination, and perception of body image.

Physical examination

A complete and thorough neurological examination must be performed in all patients with memory defects, in addition to a general physical examination.

Psychomotor testing

Psychomotor testing is a skill which is only reliable in its results when performed by those appropriately trained and experienced, and hence a referral to a psychologist will be necessary, although doctors should be familiar with the available tests. The Wechsler Adult Intelligence Scale (WAIS) generates an intelligence quotient but can indicate brain damage by discrepancies in scores between the various sub-tests. Other tests which include memory function and may be useful are the Graham Kendall Memory for Design's Test, and the Halstead-Reitan battery.

Other investigations

These should be performed as appropriate, for example an EEG and a CAT Scan.

DIFFERENTIAL DIAGNOSIS

Table 19.2 indicates the most likely diagnosis for different types of memory loss, but also shows that diagnosis depends on the association of memory dysfunction with other signs and symptoms and can rarely be made on memory alone.

MEMORY IMPAIRMENT AND PSYCHIATRIC ILLNESS

Organic psychoses

Acute confusional state (see Table 19.3)

In acute organic psychoses, memory is impaired along with other cognitive functions of perception and its assimilation. However, attention and concentration are usually seriously impaired both by clouded consciousness and preoccupation with frightening images and beliefs, and this precludes effective memory testing. The hallmark of this disorder is disorientation which fluctuates with time (see below).

Chronic organic psychoses (*dementia*) (see Table 19.4)

Alzheimer type dementia causes a general deterioration of all intellectual functions but may be so gradual as not to come to attention until some catastrophe such as a fall or a chest infection. Memory loss may be the first symptom, but this usually occurs with less specific personality changes, such as an increase in stubbornness and querulousness and a diminution of interest in surrounding people and events. Memory for recent events is always lost before long term memories; disorientation is therefore present. If personality and social skills are relatively well preserved, the recent memory loss may not be initially evident in the clinical examination especially if the patient can generalize in his or her answer rather than be required to answer specifically from his own memory. For example if asked,' How did you get to see me today? ' he may say. 'By bus' on the grounds of first principle, when in fact his daughter brought him in her car.

The first symptoms in multi-infarct dementia may be emotional and personality changes and in the rarer dementias, where cerebral atrophy is initially confined to specific areas (such as Pick's disease affecting the frontal lobes) memory loss

Table 19.2 Some associations of disorientation, memory loss and diagnosis

Orientation	Memory loss: global	Associated with	Diagnosis
Disorientation	Recent memory	Other functions intact	Korsakov's psychosis
Disorientation	Recent ± longer	Impaired consciousness, perceptual abnormalities	Acute confusion
Impairment initially slight	Initially slight	Disinhibition, coarsening of personality, impaired insight	Pick's disease
Impaired	Recent	Choreiform movements, preceding personality change, family history	Huntington's chorea
Impaired	Recent	Motor system involvement, e.g. spastic paraplegia, involuntary movements, very rapid course	Kreutzfeldt–Jacob disease
Impaired time, place	Recent	Personality and intellectual deterioration, narrowing of interest, loss of grasp	Mild/moderate dementia (Alzheimer type)
Impaired time, place	Recent	Neurological abnormalities, cerebral/systemic atherosclerosis, step-wise progression	Multi-infarct dementia
Total disorientation: time, place, person	Immediate, recent and long term	As above plus loss of language and purposeful activity	Severe ·dementia (any cause)
Orientated	Immediate loss, intact recent/long term	(e.g.) anxiety, hallucinations	Poor concentration (? cause)
Usually orientated	Recent	Depressive signs and symptoms	Depressive pseudodementia
Initially disorientated, later orientated	Recent ± past, personal events	Stressful recent event	Dissociative (hysterical) amnesia
Initially disorientated, later orientated	Recent ± past, personal events	Depressive signs and symptoms	Depressive fugue
Remains disorientated	Recent, immediate and past personal knowledge	No mental state abnormalities, identification evidence absent	Malingering, simulated amnesia

Orientation	Memory Loss: partial	Associated with	Diagnosis
Initial disorientation	All events for minutes prior to trauma	Head injury	Retrograde amnesia
Initial disorientation	All events hours or days after trauma	Head injury	Anterograde amnesia
Normal	Specific past events	Anxiety/depressive symptoms	Repression of painful memories
Normal	Non-specific, patchy inadequate memory	Chronic psychotic signs/symptoms	Chronic schizophrenia
Normal	Non-specific, patchy inadequate memory	Poor educational achievement	Low intelligence

Table 19.3 Acute organic psychoses

Clinical picture	Impairment of consciousness	
	Disorientation in time and place	} 'confusion'
	Visual & other perceptual abnormalities illusions	
	hallucinations	
	Thinking slow and muddled	

Table 19.3 (*cont'd*)

	Agitation, restlessness, and fear
	Suspicion, misunderstanding and paranoia
Causes	Systemic
	drug intoxication/withdrawal
	other toxic substances, alcohol, solvents, anaesthetic agents
	metabolic: electrolyte disturbance, uraemia, hepatic failure
	endocrine
	cardiovascular
	infection
	nutritional and vitamin deficiency
	Local
	space-occupying lesions
	post-traumatic
	cerebrovascular
	infections
	epilepsy

Table 19.4 Chronic organic psychoses

Clinical picture	Clear consciousness
	progressive loss of memory, learning and grasp
	intellectual and personality deterioration
	progressive reduction in self-care ability
	language and communication failure
	disorientation in time, place and person
Causes	Systemic
	toxic: alcohol
	endocrine: myxoedema
	anoxia: anaemia, cardiac failure
	vitamin deficiency, B, B_{12}, folic acid
	Local
	degenerative
	Alzheimer's, Pick's, Huntington's, Kreuzfeldt-Jacob, Parkinson's diseases
	vascular
	multi-infarct, single catastrophic infarct
	infection
	neurosyphilis, encephalitis
	post-traumatic
	space-occupying lesion

may be a late symptom. There is no diagnostic reliability, however, in the pattern of developing symptoms and memory is always affected at some stage, and usually early, in the disease process. Demented patients may for many years preserve memory for events predating the onset of the illness, but as the disease progresses, memory becomes reliable only for events further and further in the past. Severely demented patients may only be able to recall childhood happenings, and frequently talk about their childhood as if they were experiencing it now. In the final stages of dementia, it is impossible to test memory, since both comprehension and expression of language become too impaired.

Korsakov's psychosis (the dysmnesic syndrome) (see Table 19.5)

Loss of short term memory with complete preservation of intellect is the rule in this syndrome, which results from damage to the posterior hypothalamus, the mamillary bodies and the floor of the third ventricle. Research has shown the presence of retrograde amnesia which may last for months or years. The causes of Korsakov's psychosis are shown in Table 19.5, but the overwhelming majority of cases arisen from thiamine deficiency in alcoholism. Alcoholics frequently fail to maintain an adequate diet, both because of loss of appetite for food (for example from gastritis)

Table 19.5 Causes of Korsakov's psychosis

Thiamine deficiency:
  alcoholism

  carcinoma of stomach

  pregnancy

  malabsorption

  dietary deficiency

Tumours in:
  IIIrd ventricle

  hypothalamus

Subarachnoid haemorrhage

Bilateral posterior cerebral artery occlusion

Carbon monoxide poisoning

Tuberculous meningitis

and because they may not be able to afford food as well as drink; since their calorific intake from alcohol may be sufficient to maintain weight, developing malnutrition may not be noticed. Thiamine deficiency occurs because thiamine is depleted in carbohydrate metabolism, and Wernicke's encephalopathy results (clouding of consciousness, ataxia, nystagmus and opthalmoplegia; see Chapter 7). Upon resolution of the encephalopathy, the chronic disability of loss of short term memory becomes clear.

The clinical picture is striking. As far as retrograde amnesia allows, patients will be able to give an entirely appropriate and accurate account of events prior to the illness, and their intellectual ability is unimpaired. They will also be able to perform accurately on tests of immediate memory — for example, they will be able to repeat a name or series of numbers immediately — but will demonstrate complete inability to store this information for more than one or two seconds. The classic example is the patient who registers the doctor's name and converses with him for a while, but when the doctor leaves the room and returns a minute or so later, fails to recognize him and denies having seen him before. Disorientation is present, most particularly for time and place. Confabulation — the presentation of made up, false answers in response to questions necessitating the presence of recent memory — is one of the hallmarks of the dysmnesic syndrome, but may occur in other disorders. In Korsakov's psychosis it may be due to a number of causes, including an inability to differentiate between current reality and past memories, suggestibility and educated guesswork. In any condition, such as the early stages of dementia when insight is retained, and intellectual grasp and social skills are not impaired, patients with poor recent memory may consciously attempt to cover embarrassment by offering plausible explanations. However, in Korsakov's psychosis, the conscious element is probably much less significant than the rekindling of old memories in response to questioning. Confabulation must be distinguished from lying for gain, and should only be described in patients with organic memory impairment. A diagnostic pitfall is the failure to date the onset of the condition, since memory is preserved only before this time. For instance, a patient who has had Korsakov's psychosis for twenty years will show memory defects on both short and long term testing, wrongly suggesting a diagnosis of dementia. Patients may have had partial success from treatment to replace thiamine and show some ability to learn, especially if their environment remains reasonably constant; they may therefore become reasonably orientated to their surroundings. Another diagnostic difficulty occurs in alcoholics who, have in addition a continuing global dementia, which obscures the clinical picture.

Hippocampal lesions

A clinical picture which resembles Korsakov's psychosis results from bilateral damage to the hippocampal regions of the temporal lobes. This can result from bilateral thrombosis of the posterior cerebral artery, but in addition patients with intractable temporal lobe epilepsy have on occasion been treated by bilateral temporal lobectomy, with resulting impairment of short term memory. The condition can arise after resection of one temporal lobe if the patient has bilateral epileptic foci, indicating damage to both.

Head injury (see Chapter 10)

Head injury with loss of consciousness invariably produces memory loss which may last for seconds only, but may continue for weeks or months. Memory loss is divided into *retrograde:* the time between the moment of injury and the last clear recollection before the injury; and *anterograde* (post-traumatic:) the time between the moment of injury and resumption of normal memory. Retrograde amnesia usually lasts for a shorter period than anterograde and may only be for a matter of minutes. Very long periods of retrograde amnesia may be caused by the combination of organic damage and the emotional response to trauma.

Anterograde amnesia usually terminates abruptly with full resumption of normal memory. Its duration is of prognostic value for both intellectual impairment and psychiatric disability. Post-traumatic amnesia of less than an hour usually predicts full recovery; but if it lasts more than a week

is likely to herald continuing disability. This relationship is most apparent in closed head injuries, since in open injuries local damage in vulnerable areas of the brain may cause more severe memory impairment. Visual memory (topographical memory) for example, may be lost following damage to the parietal lobes. Chronic head injury, such as may be caused by boxing, may result in short term memory loss or global dementia.

Transient global amnesia

Transient global amnesia, first identified about twenty years ago, is a condition which occurs in middle age, affects men more than women and is probably caused by cerebrovascular disorder. As its name implies it is a self-limiting disruption of memory which occurs in clear consciousness and with no evidence of other neurological impairment. Its duration is usually several hours, during which time a retrograde amnesia occurs, together with disorientation and loss of immediate memory, but with preservation of past events and knowledge of individual identity and circumstances. Upon recovery, amnesia for the period persists.

FUNCTIONAL PSYCHOSES

Major depression

Apparent memory loss is a common symptom in severe depression (depressive pseudodementia) and results from failure of registration due to poor concentration and attention. Clinical testing in such patients reveals poor immediate memory, but if the patient can be persuaded to concentrate on the task, memory functions will be found to be unimpaired. Depressive pseudodementia is more common in the elderly and may reflect a lack of cerebral reserve. In some elderly patients, memory loss will be identifiable on testing or may persist after the depression has recovered; in these a coexisting dementia will be discovered although this diagnosis may only be made in retrospect. An important indicator in the differentiation of depression and dementia in the elderly is that in the former, memory may appear to be affected but orientation remains relatively unimpaired. Disorientation, on the other hand, is prominent in dementia.

Mania

Manic patients will not normally complain of loss of any ability, including memory, but may demonstrate apparent memory loss due to registration failure. They are not co-operative in memory testing and their failure to recall recent events results from their preoccupation and distractibility.

Schizophrenia

Acute schizophrenia results in a picture similar to that in mania; the acutely psychotic patient may be too preoccupied to record normal everyday events, although his memory for events of emotional significance, for example those which have been incorporated into a delusional system, remains unimpaired.

Chronic schizophrenic patients, because of isolation, withdrawal and apathy, may demonstrate a generalized patchy memory loss for past personal events and general information. Memory testing may be very difficult in the presence of thought disorder. Recent evidence of cerebral atrophy in some series of chronic schizophrenic patients suggests that the organic defect in this disease may be greater than hitherto supposed; this interesting question remains unresolved.

NEUROSIS

Anxiety, depression and obsessional states

Patients with these states frequently closely monitor their own functioning and may complain of poor memory. As in the functional psychoses, registration and recall are affected by these conditions, and patients act absentmindedly and fail to concentrate on the matter in hand. Heightened levels of arousal in anxiety states may result in an excess of sensory input with a relative failure to select significant items for memory storage.

Partial loss of memory for past personal events occurs in neurotic conditions as a result of psychological problems associated with the period in question. For example, a patient who had no memory of her father's desertion of the family when she was aged six, had repressed both the event and her feelings at the time in order to avoid pain and conflict. Similary, exceptional stress such as occurs in disasters or battle may result in partial dissociation from some exceptionally painful aspects of the occasion. The patient will normally remember being involved in the situation but have little or no memory of its detail.

Global loss of memory

Total loss of memory is found, rarely, in hysterical dissociative states. Patients with amnesia of this type are frequently found wandering in fugue states with, apparently, no awareness of identity or of past or recent events. Reasoning ability, language, new learning ability and self-care are unimpaired, which makes the distinction between psychogenic and severe organic amnesias a simple one. Simulation may be suspected if the patient fails to recall anything, even immediately, on memory testing, and simulation is also likely when evidence of personal identity has carefully been removed from clothing and handbags. Psychogenic amnesias are a response to intolerable stress in a person's life, and may be precipitated by a devastating threat to self-esteem, for example financial ruin. Potential criminal proceedings are not uncommon in such patients which again raises the suspicion of malingering.

Differential diagnosis can, rarely, become extremely complicated when the precipitating stress has been a development of an organic dementia and the two conditions coexist.

DISORDERS OF ORIENTATION

The integration of input from the special senses with memory and judgement to provide a constant awareness of one's surroundings is a basic cognitive task which we take for granted. Those handicapped by subnormal intelligence, especially the severely subnormal, may never fully achieve orientation in time and place although they will usually recognize their name. Clearly, abnormalities in orientation in previously normal people denote abnormal cerebral function.

Disorientation is usually considered in respect of orientation for time, place and person. *Temporal* orientation is normally quite precise: the approximate time of day is known, and certainly whether it is morning, afternoon or evening; and the day of the week, month and year should be known without any difficulty. The date of the month is less reliable and there is a *caveat* regarding people in institutions such as hospital or prisons about the day of the week, since it is difficult to discriminate between days when one is much the same as the next. *Spatial* orientation should again be precisely known, assuming that the person has been in his surroundings for a sufficiently long period of time. Hence a person should immediately identify the room of his house which he is in, its address, town, relationships to shops, post boxes etc. Orientation *for person* is tested by asking the person his name, and the identity of other, known persons.

Impairment of orientation usually proceeds with severity, from impairment of time, through place, and finally to person.

The ability to orientate depends on :

1 intact sensory input

2 preservation of all memory functions; registration, retention, recognition and recall, so that incoming sensory signals can be tested against past experience

3 integrity of higher intellectual function so that new evidence can be integrated and hypotheses generated and tested.

Disturbances of orientation may involve one or more of these functions.

Loss of special sensation, such as sudden blindness, will result in disorientation, most especially in this case for place, until the person learns to use other senses, such as touch and hearing, to compensate.

Disorientation can be induced, usually for experimental purposes, by placing subjects in conditions where the special senses are deprived of stimuli. Subjects placed in soundproof, empty, dark chambers will quickly lose orientation for time.

Where short term memory is largely or completely absent the patient will be unable to tell the time and will not recognize his surroundings unless he is in a very familiar place which is stored in his long term memory. He will, however, be able to use his intellect to deduce the kind of place he is in: for example to recognize a room with a cooker, sink and fridge as a kitchen, without being able to locate in whose house the room is.

The most frequent causes of disorientation in clinical practice, however, involve disturbances in all three functions.

Acute organic psychoses

Disorientation in acute organic psychosis (delirium), invariably involves sensory input disturbance as well as other cognitive impairment, because the clouding of consciousness pathognomonic of acute confusion interrupts the inflow and processing of information from external senses. Internal messages from disturbed memory and thinking (similar to dreams) may be interpreted as if they were external sensations, thus producing the misperceptions, hallucinations and delusions common in this condition. Disorientation is usually of time and place and will fluctuate with the impairment of consciousness. Thus, the patient may be quite disorientated at one time but may be completely lucid an hour or so later.

Chronic organic psychoses

Chronic organic psychosis (dementia) causes disorientation principally because of progressive failure of intellect, grasp and memory, although perception is involved as the dementing process relentlessly destroys all cerebral function. Consciousness is clear in this condition and the patient may be bright, alert and apparently functioning reasonably well. Temporal disorientation in clear consciousness should always give rise to investigation for dementia.

Commonly, the first sign of such a process is the person wandering, lost, in the street, intent on doing the shopping at 2 am. Short term memory is impaired first in dementia, but the more severe the condition, the more likely it is that long term memory failure will add to the disorientation. In a severe case, the person will fail to recognize the house she has lived in for fifty years as her own, and may refer to herself by her maiden name, or may not be able either to say, or to recognize, her first name.

Functional psychoses

Patients with a functional psychosis may interpret their surroundings delusionally; for example, the patient who claimed that the women's hostel in which she was staying was, in fact, her house. Further questioning revealed her knowledge that everyone else believed this building to be a hostel, and she had no doubt of its address; only she, however, knew that the order of nuns in charge of the hostel had illegally dispossessed her and that she was the rightful owner.

CONFUSION

This ordinary word has been adopted and redefined by psychiatrists in a very specific sense to indicate the presence of clouding of consciousness and disorientation in acute cerebral dysfunction. It also continues to be used, however, in its original general sense to denote difficulty in thinking and the mixture of different themes and elements in thought arising from any cause; and this gives rise to problems in usage. It is probably best to avoid the word entirely in a technical sense when describing the mental state of the patient. If, however, it is used, it should be restricted to its organic sense, and other words such as bewilderment and perplexity should be used in describing other types of thought disorder.

PERPLEXITY

Perplexity is the name given to the state of bewildered incomprehension characteristically found in acute schizophrenia. It results from increased arousal together with conflicting thoughts, beliefs and suspicions as the patient attempts to order his thoughts in a way that he can comprehend.

CASE HISTORY

MARTIN PARKER

Martin Parker was a 65-year-old self-employed accountant who was referred by his general practitioner for a psychiatric opinion with a complaint that he was unable to concentrate at work as well as he used to. He first became aware of this when he noticed himself making mistakes while auditing clients' books. Because of this he had taken to checking his work three times rather than his usual twice. He also mentioned that on a couple of occasions he had mislaid files he had been dealing with and was finding it increasingly difficult to remember names.

On further questioning he admitted that the last two years had been extremely worrying: his wife had been very ill with cancer; his business had been doing badly and his younger son had been involved with drugs. He said that at times he felt very tense, was smoking more and often needed a drink when he came home in the evening to help him unwind. For the last three months he had been having difficulty getting off to sleep, no longer enjoyed playing bridge or golf and had generally lost his zest for life. He had always been fairly sociable but recently he had to push himself to go out. However, his appetite and weight were unchanged and there had been no alteration in his sexual habits.

His father, a successful accountant who had started the firm of which Mr Parker was the senior partner, was a stern and rigid man, unable to show affection. He had become senile in his mid-sixties after which he had lingered on for five years having to be cared for by his wife — 'a fate worse than death' said Martin Parker. His mother was an overweight, affectionate lady who tended to smother her son, perhaps as a response to the death of his only sibling from the effects of an accident one year before Martin was born. There was no other relevant family history.

He had been a timid, frightened child; he had

found it difficult to settle into boarding school and had spend many a night crying himself to sleep. However, he was good at cricket and gradually made a circle of friends. He did well in his examinations and went to Oxford where he got a first class degree in economics. He then entered his father's business. Initially Martin found it difficult being the son of the boss, because his father set him virtually impossible standards and he would often come home from work in the evening absolutely drained.

In his late twenties he met Cynthia, a doctor's daughter, and a year later they got married. Their marriage had been, and was still by all accounts, a happy one although Martin found it difficult to show affection to his three sons and one daughter. In keeping with this he said he had never been able to show his feelings which he kept bottled up and this was confirmed by his wife. She also said that he had been a perfectionist who frequently stayed late at the office to finish his work, which he would never consider leaving to the next day. His office was always meticulously tidy and he became very upset if any of his things were moved.

He had suffered for some twenty years with an irritable bowel which caused problems whenever he was under stress. Over the last two years and particularly the last six months it had become especially bad. Prior to the last year or two he had drunk very little and then only at mealtimes or social occasions, and he had confined his smoking to the occasional cigar. As noted above these habits had recently changed.

At interview Mr Parker looked tense and was continually shifting around in his chair. He found it very difficult to talk about personal and private matters but the form of his speech was normal. He admitted to being anxious and unhappy but there were no suicidal thoughts, delusions or hallucinations. He was fully orientated but had difficulty remembering a name and address after three minutes, and there were surprising gaps in his knowledge of current affairs.

His wife confirmed the story of change in her husband over the last three years. She said that he had forgotten to come home in time for a dinner party they held for friends, and he had also

for the first time in their marriage failed to send her an anniversary card. He was now having to make lists of important pieces of information and he carried these lists around in his diary.

Questions

What diagnoses would fit the symptoms and signs?
How would you investigate the situation further to clarify the diagnosis?

Mr Parker has an obsessional personality. Superimposed upon this a change in mood has developed, with anxiety and depression and a deterioration in his intellectual capacity. The possible diagnoses are of an anxiety state, a depressive illness, a dementing process or a combination of these. The intellectual impairment may be merely due to a lack of attention and concentration consequent on either increased anxiety or depression — a pseudodementia.

The symptoms in favour of an anxiety state are Mr Parker's subjective feelings of being tense, borne out on objective examination, the worsening of his irritable bowel, his increased smoking and drinking and his difficulty getting off to sleep. In addition his symptoms have occurred at a time when he has been under considerable stress.

Depression would account for his loss of interest, social withdrawal and feelings of unhappiness. However the lack of change in appetite, weight and sexual drive, and the fact that the change in sleep is in a direction of difficulty getting off to sleep rather than early morning waking is against the diagnosis of a major depressive syndrome. Therefore if one were to say he was pathologically depressed the diagnosis would be depressive neurosis or dysthymic disorder.

The only symptoms which would lead one to diagnose a dementing process are intellectual impairment and a family history of dementia. As he is now only sixty-five and the symptoms have come on over the last two years the diagnosis would be pre-senile dementia with depression and anxiety secondary to this, due both to his awareness of his failing intellect and to his difficulty in coping at work.

Mr Parker needs a full cognitive assessment

including testing of higher cortical centres and the use of a brief standardized questionnaire. Laboratory investigations may reveal a systemic cause for his intellectual impairment and an EEG and CAT scan may also be helpful. Full psychological tests may help to distinguish between dementia and pseudodementia but this is not foolproof. Serial psychometry will show any deterioration due to dementia, or improvement with treatment of a mood disorder. Admission to hospital for assessment of mood and behaviour might be useful and might also provide an opportunity to assess intellect in a controlled, stress-free atmosphere. In some cases, however, the diagnosis can only be made in retrospect, based on the subsequent history of the disorder.

20

Episodic disturbances of consciousness — 'Funny turns'

Attacks of altered awareness or behaviour are commonly complained of by patients and their differential diagnosis can be a complex and lengthy process. The patient should be asked fully to describe the phenomena and a detailed psychiatric and physical history and examination should be carried out. Generally patients are complaining of short-lived episodes, of sudden onset and rapid and complete recovery, over which they have no control. They usually experience changes in consciousness together with a complex of other symptoms. The first task is to determine whether or not a clearly defined episode of abnormality is indeed occurring. Many people express uncharacteristic and/or uncontrolled emotional outbursts in terms reminiscent of an attack: 'I don't know what comes over me — I can't help myself'; especially if the behaviour is aggressive, dishonest or otherwise antisocial, or if it is apparently linked to physiological effects as in the pre-menstruum. This initial discrimination is rarely difficult.

Neither should it be difficult to differentiate episodic phenomena from continuous states of changed consciousness, whether or not within this change there are fluctuations in severity and extent. Changes in consciousness over periods of days or longer which do not spontaneously recover are not considered here but in Chapter 19. Similarly, stuporose conditions in which some aspects of consciousness are preserved, and which do not fall within the spectrum between alert states and coma, are considered in Chapter 3; alterations in consciousness as a disturbance of the continuum between wakefulness and sleep are discussed in Chapter 5. We are left, then, with the differential diagnosis of conditions in which there is a specific history of sudden onset of changed consciousness from minor alteration to loss of consciousness; with a duration of minutes, or more rarely hours; with rapid or gradual, but complete, recovery; which may or may not be linked to identified triggers or specific times of day; and is of variable or predictable frequency. A complete account of a typical attack, both as subjectively experienced and as objectively observed, is essential to diagnosis. The total clinical picture, including the age of the patient and concurrent physical and psychiatric diagnosis, will indicate the most likely of the many causes.

Most of these conditions can be described as fits, faints or falls, although complaints of other symptoms, such as dizziness, may pre-dominate (see Table 20.1).

FAINTING

Cerebral hypoxia and/or hypoglycaemia leads to the characteristic pattern of the syncopal attack: an onset over several seconds of a feeling of distance, nausea, and restriction of vision, followed by loss of consciousness, and falling. In benign syncope, cerebral perfusion is rapidly re-established by increase in cardiac output, and consciousness returns to complete normality within a few minutes. Common physiological causes are reduced cardiac output due to venous pooling on immobile standing, especially in hot weather with associated vasodilation; fatigue; hunger; and pregnancy. It also occurs commonly in adolescent girls, especially around menstruation; with sudden postural change, especially in the elderly; and occasionally after prolonged bouts of coughing. Simple syncope is invariably related

Table 20.1 Typical pattern of attack disorders

	Before attack	During	After
Simple syncope	Nausea, sweating	Consciousness lost, bradycardia	Quick recovery
Panic attacks	Hyperventilation, anxiety	Paraesthesia, sweating, tetany, change in consciousness	Gradual complete recovery
Cardiac arrhythmias/ cerebrovascular disease	No warning	Sudden loss of consciousness	Sudden recovery
Epilepsy	Aura, or no warning	*Grand mal:* Unconsciousness, tonic/clonic spasm incontinence *Petit mal:* 'absence' *Psychomotor* Apparently conscious but uncommunicative; semi-purposeful behaviour	Slow recovery, sleepiness, confusion
Non-epileptic fits	Dramatic scream/cry or other behaviour	Apparent unconsciousness but responsive; bizarre, purposeful asymnetic activity; injury rare	Variable: slow, dramatic, or quick and complete

to posture and its occurrence in patients whilst sitting or lying down indicates pathological disturbance of cerebral oxygenation.

The most frequent psychological cause of fainting is anxiety, especially during hyperventilation attacks (see Chapter 13).

Hyperventilation results in hypocapnia, which causes cerebral vasoconstriction and anoxia. The physiological effects of hyperventilation are legion and include paraesthaesia and tetany in addition to a sensation of breathlessness, tachycardia and nausea. Most commonly patients hyperventilating in a panic attack experience the prodromal features of syncope without losing consciousness; but the resulting fear of fainting exacerbates the anxiety state, and is frequently expressed by patients whose anxiety attacks are phobic — for example, fear of fainting in supermarkets.

When depersonalization occurs in the context of hyperventilation it is experienced episodically and may indeed be the principal symptom. Care must be taken to distinguish such attacks from epilepsy, by careful elucidation of diagnostic features of the anxiety and panic. Depersonalization is the experience of alteration of the sense of self, and is frequently associated with derealization, where the environment is experienced as flat, unreal or remote. It is characteristically an unpleasant experience and patients will describe feeling cut-off, remote and unnatural; sometimes they feel as if their appearance changes.

It is essential to obtain the 'as if' quality from the patient; depersonalization is an abnormality not of belief but of perception; and the patient knows that in reality neither he nor the rest of the world is changed.

The diagnosis of anxiety states as a cause of episodic alteration in consciousness not only depends on the nature of the attack as described above, but may be further supported by establishing the presence either of a generalized or a phobic anxiety state. The cause of the anxiety must be established and the whole clinical picture will be necessary to the diagnosis.

Diagnostic confusion may arise when cardiovascular, cerebrovascular or other systemic causes of faints and falls coexist with anxiety. Not only are anxiety states no protection against physical disease, but patients who intermittently lose consciousness become anxious about it and are thus prone to the same cycle of reinforcing symptoms as described above. Attacks of recent onset in middle-aged and elderly people are most likely to be due to cardiovascular (myocardial infarct, arrhytmias) of cerebrovascular (transient ischaemic attacks, carotid or vertebrobasilar insufficiency) pathology.

Paroxysmal cardiac arrhythmias may be wrongly diagnosed as panic attacks, especially in young adults where other clinical signs may be absent. Fast tachycardia, or bradycardia, during the attack, which is terminated by an abrupt change in pulse rate; is suggestive of arrhythmia and must be excluded by an ECG taken during an attack. It is essential to exclude hypoglycaemia as a cause of attacks of altered consciousness. Hypoglycaemia may present as changed, disinhibited behaviour, usually following a feeling of faintness and nausea with progress to ataxia and drowsiness and loss of consciousness, with or without epileptic fits. It is important to bear in mind the possibility of self-limiting hypoglycaemia, due to insulinoma or excessive insulin response to glucose, drugs or alcohol, and blood sugar estimations at the outset of the attack should be performed.

FALLS

Complaints of falling to the ground without noticeable loss of consciousness are commonest in elderly patients where vertebrobasilar insufficiency or cardiac conduction defects (for example Stokes-Adams attacks) must be suspected. However, for many elderly people, a generalized frailty, with impaired eyesight and balance, is sufficient to produce falling; often with disastrous consequences for elderly osteoporotic femurs. In younger people, falling may similarly be caused by organic illness; as a result of neurological disease causing weakness; visual impairment; or vestibular disease (where falling to the ground is preceded by vertigo, for example in Menière's disease). Falling may be a psychiatric symptom: a feature of anxiety or panic attacks, or a histrionic display of illness in an attention-seeking patient. Falling also occurs as a true hysterical symptom

(see below) although a more complex attack with features other than simple falling is the rule in hysterical seizures. Cataplexy (see Chapter 3) is a rare but important cause of falling due to sudden loss of muscle tone.

FITS

Differential Diagnosis

A fit is generally considered to be the combination of loss of consciousness and involuntary convulsive muscular spasm. The most import differential diagnosis lies between epileptic and non-epileptic fits, and although the natural history and associated observations of the attack may be adequate discriminators, electroencephalographic (EEG) evident obtained during the attack is sometimes the only sure method of diagnosis. Patients with fits fall into one of three categories: 1 those whose fits are always epileptic; 2 those whose fits are never epileptic; and 3 those epileptic patients who sometimes have additional non-epileptic fits.

The clinical diagnosis of epilepsy is often dependent on the observations of witnesses to the attack, although the patient's history of aura (which is usually stereotyped) and post-ictal disorientation and sleepiness, together with transient abnormal neurological signs, such as an extensor plantar response, may indicate a diagnosis of epilepsy. The combination of unconsciousness, tonic and clonic muscle spasm, incontinence, tongue-biting, cyanosis and injury to limbs during clonic convulsion is invaluable clinical evidence of epilepsy, and further investigation may be necessary only to distinguish its type and to identify its cause. Conversely true tonic-clonic epilepsy is unlikely as a cause if the witnesses of a fit report no true unconsciousness (for example, talking or screaming during the attack although the patient is apparently unrousable), together with generalized bilateral thrashing of limbs rather than identifiable tonic and clonic phases; a degree of purposeful behaviour may be described. Incontinence and tongue-biting are rare in non-epileptic fits. Non-epileptic attacks are also more likely if each fit is different in its form, its antecedents and its manner and speed of recovery.

The classical differential diagnosis of non-epileptic fits has hysteria heading the list. This diagnosis must be made with extreme care, in this context as in all forms of conversion hysteria. It should not be made without other pointers, such as evidence of primary as well as secondary gain, although firm evidence of primary gain may be very difficult to establish in the assessment period, since the patient is by definition unconscious of it. The combination of fits with other current or past history of hysterical conversion is helpful. Fits are said to be a common complaint in Briquet's hysteria — an exclusively female complaint where repeated investigation and intervention for somatic complaints is the rule (see Chapter 21).

If there is evidence of conscious simulation of fits, malingering, rather than hysteria, should be the diagnosis. Panic attacks with hyperventilation may present as fits, usually in patients with anxiety or agitated depression. Hyperventilation may induce true epileptic fits in patients with low convulsive thresholds.

Diagnostic difficulties arise, however, when a patient's fits are not typical, have some epileptic and some non-epileptic features, are of more than one type, or on occasion appear to be precipitated by stress. Focal or psychomotor (that is, where ictal activity results in behavioural change rather than convulsions) fits may be particularly difficult to diagnose, especially if the aura is bizarre and complex (see below). Epileptic fits can be and often are precipitated by anger or distress, and patients with epilepsy may have fits of more than one type. However, true epilepsy is not only no protection from non-epileptic fits, but can, in some individuals, increase the likelihood of pseudo-fits by providing an experience which can be learned from. Epilepsy is disabling and stigmatizing and can have serious consequences for education, employment and social development, but the occurrence of a fit at a particular time may create a climate whereby responsibilities or unpleasant tasks are seen to be avoided by its timing. Some epileptic patients therefore may have a combination of epileptic and non-epileptic attacks, and these must be discriminated if appropriate treatment is to ensue.

Developments in EEG technology have improved diagnostic accuracy in this group (see Table 20.2). All generalized epileptic attacks will show EEG abnormalities of spikes and waves before, during or after the attack, and some patients will show constant EEG abnormalities. However, many epileptic patients have normal EEGs between attacks, although the time taken for the EEG to normalize varies between individuals. The only types of epilepsy which are consistent with a normal EEG taken by surface electrodes are focal forms where the lesions are small and discrete. Sphenoidal leads may be necessary for a diagnosis of complex partial epilepsy. Non-epileptic patients may have non-specific EEG abnormalities, which are not infrequent in the general population; but these abnormalities will not change during an attack. Ambulatory monitoring of EEG activity may be a necessary final arbiter of the diagnosis, but even then can only be conclusive when all the known types of attack have been monitored.

A fourth category of fits must finally be considered: those patients who have epileptic attacks which are drug-related. An important group is epileptics whose anticonvulsant medication has been changed or increased. An increase in fit frequency may follow anticonvulsant toxicity or withdrawal. Epileptic fits can be precipitated by the administration of neuroleptics or tricyclic antidepressants, by the sudden cessation of benzodiazepines, by both the administration and sudden cessation of barbiturates, and by the abuse of drugs such as alcohol or solvents. A careful history of drug use (prescribed, 'borrowed' or illicit) and

Table 20.2 Attacks

	EEG: Between attacks	EEG: During attacks
Epileptic	30% normal or nonspecific 70% spikes and waves	Abnormal (may be obscured by muscle artefact)
Non-epileptic	Normal or nonspecific	Normal or nonspecific
Epileptic and non-epileptic	Normal/abnormal	Abnormal and normal

changes in use is essential in the investigation of attack disorders.

Complex-Partial (Temporal Lobe) Epilepsy

Epilepsy has, for centuries, been a much feared and troublesome disorder, causing attacks of altered or lost consciousness. There are many different varieties of epilepsy but it can be classified under two main headings: those in which the epileptic discharge is generalized (this includes types previously known as grand mal and petit mal) and those in which there is a partial onset from a cerebral focus (including psychomotor or temporal lobe discharge; see Table 20.3). Full discussion of the diagnosis of epilepsy is beyond the remit of this book, but as Sherrington said,'The Sylvian fissure divides neurology from psychiatry' and it is true, in clinical practice, that complex partial (temporal lobe) seizures may present initially to the psychiatrist since their neurological origin may be difficult to establish.

Table 20.3 Classification of epilepsy

Current terminology	Previous terminology
Generalized	
epilepsy: primary	
secondary	
tonic-clonic	grandmal
absences	petit mal
akinetic	akinetic
Partial (focal)	
epilepsy: complex	temporal lobe psychomotor
elementary	e.g. Jacksonian

A diagnostic problem in complex partial epilepsy may occur when the focal seizure is not generalized to the centrencephalus to produce a classic tonic-clonic fit, but to the limbic system (psychomotor attack). In this case, the patient may be able to carry out complicated, apparently purposeful behaviour, although his consciousness is impaired and he will be largely inaccessible during the attack.

The ictal phase

The *aura* occurs at the onset of the abnormal electrical discharge and is experienced by the patient before he loses consciousness. The presence of an aura denotes epilepsy of focal origin and its type may be useful for localization. It should be distinguished from the prodromal stage of epilepsy, which is not ictal but precedes the attack in some individuals. Prodromata may continue for hours or days and are usually mental changes such as irritability, lethargy or anxiety which are terminated by the fit.

Auras which originate in the temporal lobe are autonomic, perceptual, cognitive or affective in type (see Table 20.4). All of these may lead to a misdiagnosis of psychiatric disease, especially the perceptual auras which may give rise to a wrong diagnosis of functional psychosis, and autonomic ones which may be difficult to differentiate from anxiety states. However, although it may be difficult for the patient to describe the aura, it is usually stereotyped and a different experience from anything else, such as anxiety felt at other times by the patient. The differential diagnosis should not be difficult when the attack is generalized to a tonic-clonic fit, but may be if the attack is psychomotor in type, especially when this part of the seizure is relatively brief. It is always essential to obtain a full history from the patient and other informants of the circumstances surrounding the aura, so that the presence of automatic behaviour can be identified. Some patients continue what they are doing although they are evidently preoccupied and do not respond coherently when spoken to. Others perform different, sometimes

Table 20.4 Temporal lobe auras

Autonomic	epigastric 'butterflies' or churning in stomach tachycardia, apnoea flushing, pallor
Perceptual	Déjà vu, jamais vu visual, olfactory, gustatory or auditory hallucinations micropsia, macropsia
Cognitive	dysphasia memory disturbance incoherent thinking
Affective	anxiety, fear depression, anger

complex, tasks like making a cup of tea, but most automatic behaviour is non-specific, like getting up and wandering around the room. Diagnosis is aided in those patients in whom the automatic behaviour is itself sterotyped.

Post-ictal phase

Psychomotor seizures usually last for a few minutes, although serial or status attacks may lead to a duration of hours. The patient is amnesic for the attack, apart from the aura, and, as in generalized epilepsy, will usually feel drowsy and fall asleep; but in some patients a post-ictal state of confusion and irritability occurs. Post-ictal automatic behaviour is frequent in some patients. It is usually of short duration, aimless and unproductive, and, sometimes stereotyped. Automatic behaviour can, rarely, be violent although this has been overstressed. Patients may indeed react aggressively, fearfully or irritably when approached, but motivated, competent acts of aggression are rare.

Epileptic fugues are uncommon, and consist of altered behaviour over a longer period of time such as hours or days. They often involve the patient wandering from home, are post-ictal rather than ictal, and may be strongly influenced by psychological factors.

Inter-ictal states

Most patients with epilepsy lead virtually normal lives between attacks but many factors operate to determine the quality of life. These include fit frequency, the control of unwanted or toxic effects of medication, the individual personality, family and social structure and the extent to which the patient is affected by a reduction in employment prospects, social life and interests consequent upon his epilepsy. The concept of the epileptic personality as a unified type is no longer held, but it is true that there is a higher than expected incidence of personality disorders amongst epileptics; there is for example an increased prevalence of epilepsy among the prison population.

Some abnormal behaviours and moods, for example increased irritability, may be accounted for in the inter-ictal phase by continuing abnormal electrical discharge, which disrupts neurophysiology but is not sufficient to provoke a seizure.

Psychiatric complications of complex-partial epilepsy

Personality problems are the commonest difficulty, as mentioned above, and these can be exacerbated by brain damage. Brain damage may result both from anoxia during attacks and from head injuries caused when the patient falls. Epilepsy with early onset and poor control may lead to cognitive impairment, which disrupts education.

Psychotic disorders have long been known to be associated with complex partial epilepsy, usually developing many years after onset. Schizophrenia-like psychoses are the best described but manic-depressive psychosis also occurs with increased frequency. Schizophrenia-like psychoses may be associated with lesions in the dominant temporal lobe, affective psychoses with lesions in the non-dominant. It is suggested that psychotic episodes are commoner during periods when fits are well controlled.

Neurotic disorders may develop. Phobic states, usually related to travelling or to social situations, are not uncommon. Sexual disorders are very common in complex partial epilepsy, most frequently taking the form of a reduction in sexual activity. This may, in part, be a reflection of social isolation and lack of opportunity to develop intimate relationships, but there is also evidence that lack of sexual drive and reduction in performance occur frequently in patients with long term sexual relationships.

CASE HISTORY

MR CHRISTOPHER JORDAN

Mr Christopher Jordan is a 42-year-old recently divorced man who presented at the Department of Psychiatry with a one year history of 'attacks' during which he suffered from severe headaches, nausea and occasional vomiting and dizziness. On one occasion he had fallen downstairs, after which he had been unconscious for some minutes. There was no evidence of incontinence or tongue-biting during any of the attacks. Some of them were preceded by breathlessness and paraesthesiae in his hands and feet. He had also noted some loss of hearing. Because of these symptoms he was finding it increasingly difficult to cope at work as a teacher in a secondary school. He had associated symptoms of depressed and anxious mood and difficulty getting off to sleep. He had even thought that life was not worth living.

His general practitioner had referred him for an otological opinion, and Menière's disease was diagnosed. Because of his depression and anxiety he had been prescribed antidepressants and minor tranquillizers; but he had taken them irregularly, and had at times increased the dose considerably, without deriving any lasting benefit from them.

There was no relevant family history and his childhood had been normal and happy. After leaving school he went to university and he had obtained a teaching diploma. He had been at this present job for fifteen years and had coped well despite having been involved five years previously in a road accident in which he had sustained a head injury. He was popular and well-liked both by pupils and fellow teachers, and had a busy and active social life. Three years prior to the onset of his symptoms he had had an affair with a teacher at another school whom he met at a weekend conference. This had lasted sporadically for about six months until his wife found out about it and promptly left the marital home with their three children. Despite many attempts at reconciliation she had been unwilling to return home and had instituted divorce proceedings. These had been acrimonious where they touched on the custody of the children. Because of the stress associated with this Mr Jordan had started to drink heavily and admitted to the occasional day off school. After advice from his family doctor and pressure from the headmaster he had cut down his alcohol intake considerably but there were lingering suspicions that he went on occasional drinking bouts.

At interview there was evidence of unhappiness and anxiety which he related to his symptoms. There was no evidence of delusions or hallucinations. Physical examination was normal. He was therefore admitted to hospital for further investigations to clarify the diagnosis.

Questions

What is the differential diagnosis of the attacks?
If during Mr Jordan's admission an EEG was done which showed features suggestive of epilepsy, what aetiological factors might be incriminated in this particular patient?
What is the link between depression and epilepsy?

Though Mr Jordan has Menière's disease this would only account for the dizziness, nausea, vomiting and hearing loss. Neither severe headaches nor unconsciousness are recognized features of this disorder. Mr Jordan is an anxious man and epilepsy may be precipitated by hyperventilation in susceptible patients; apparent loss of hearing and consciousness may be hysterical features related to anxiety; and headache, dizziness, nausea and vomiting are common physical accompaniments of anxiety.

Alternatively, the headache might be migrainous in nature and the nausea, vomiting, dizziness and unconsciousness may be related to this. Migraine may be precipitated by stress and may follow hyperventilation, and it has been suggested that there may be an increased incidence of epilepsy in affected individuals. The important differential as far as the headaches are concerned is from tension headaches and this may present difficulties where the two coexist or where the migraine is precipitated by stress. However, as compared to tension headaches, migraine is usually unilateral, throbbing in nature, preceded by prodromata in the majority of cases and more often associated with vomiting and visual perceptual changes. The usual frequency of attacks is much less than with tension headaches, and affected individuals commonly have a family history of migraine.

As mentioned above, migraine and epilepsy may coexist and it may occasionally be difficult to decide whether an attack is migrainous or epileptic in nature. Factors favouring migraine are a gradual loss of consciousness which is less profound; the presence of a severe headache prior to the loss of consciousness; visual phenomena and bilateral paraesthesiae. In order to delineate the diagnosis further it would be important to carry out an EEG and to try to interview an informant who had witnessed one of these attacks. Obviously if an attack should occur during his admission to hospital at a time when it is witnessed by a member of staff, observations should be written down clearly and in detail. Finally, attacks may be due to cardiovascular or metabolic disorders and these should be looked for by appropriate investigations, as multiple pathology may occur in any one patient. Finally it must be remembered that epileptic and nonepileptic attacks may coexist in the same patient.

Mr Jordan has suffered from two head injuries, one following a road accident four years prior to the onset of these attacks, and the other after falling downstairs during one of the attacks. Though most epileptic attacks following head injury have their onset within four years of the injury the onset is after this period of time in twenty-five per cent of patients. As mentioned above, hyperventilation may induce fits in people with lowered epileptic thresholds, and fit frequency may increase at times of stress. Sudden withdrawal of alcohol and/or minor tranquillizers, as may have occurred here, may lead to fits, as may large doses of some antidepressants.

It has been suggested that temporal lobe brain damage is associated with the affective psychoses. In addition epilepsy is a disabling disorder which leads to severe social consequences which may themselves lead to depression. Furthermore suicide is more common in epileptics than in the general population. However there is no evidence from controlled studies that patients with epilepsy are more likely to suffer with depression than patients with other chronic disabling disorders. Medication which might be prescribed for depressed patients or alcohol which may be abused by them can be associated with epilepsy, and anticonvulsants may in their turn lead to depression. Finally stressful life events may precipitate epilepsy and depression independently in the same patient.

21

Emotional disturbance and physical symptoms

INTRODUCTION

Psychiatric illness and physical symptoms may coexist in an individual in a number of ways. The physical symptoms may be primary due to organic pathology with the psychiatric illness secondary; the latter may be primary and present with physical symptoms; the physical symptoms may be caused by both physical and psychological factors acting together — the current concept of the term psychosomatic (see below); and physical and psychiatric illness may coexist but be unrelated. However, given the mutual interdependence between body and mind, which entails numerous feedback loops in the system, the above scheme obviously represents a gross oversimplification. Nevertheless it is a useful paradigm with which to approach an area abounding with confusion.

Diagnostic categories are often confused with aetiology: for example the multiple roles of anxiety in the production of and response to physical symptoms and illness (see Figure 4). Understandable affective reactions to illness and treatment may be seen as pathological, often due more to the observer's bias and the patient's surroundings than to mental state, lending support to the definition of a disturbed patient as one who is disturbing to those looking after him.

Despite much psychological research, little account is taken of illness behaviour, which determines the individual clinical presentation. This is dependent, not only on the patient's mental state, personality and past experiences, but also on the unwanted effects of medication and physical treatment, the relationship between the caring staff and the patient, the nature of investigations and the treatment surroundings. It is when illness behaviour diverges significantly from expected norms that a strong psychological component to the problem should be suspected: for example, a patient who remains in a dependent sick role, originally appropriate to his physical condition, long after this has resolved. Perhaps a sign of the lack of clarity which pervades our understanding and conceptualization of this area is the confusion which reigns in the terminology used. Hysteria means different things to different people; hypochondriasis is both a symptom and a diagnosis; and anxiety is often used as an umbrella term. An attempt has been made in this chapter to lay down operational guidelines for these terms as used in DSM-III.

In addition, other terms such as functional, psychogenic, psychosocial and psychosomatic, are often wrongly used or considered interchangeable, leading to further confusion in diagnosis, research and communication. It would be most helpful to keep the term 'functional' for those symptoms which are due to disturbance of function regardless of aetiology; 'psychogenic' for situations where there is an obvious psychological aetiology; 'psychosocial' for conditions where psychological and social factors are important; and 'psychosomatic' for the broad concept of interaction between organic and psychosocial factors in any given situation. The latter embraces the holistic approach of causation of illness: namely that in any disease, organic, psychological and social factors may be to some extent involved in the aetiology.

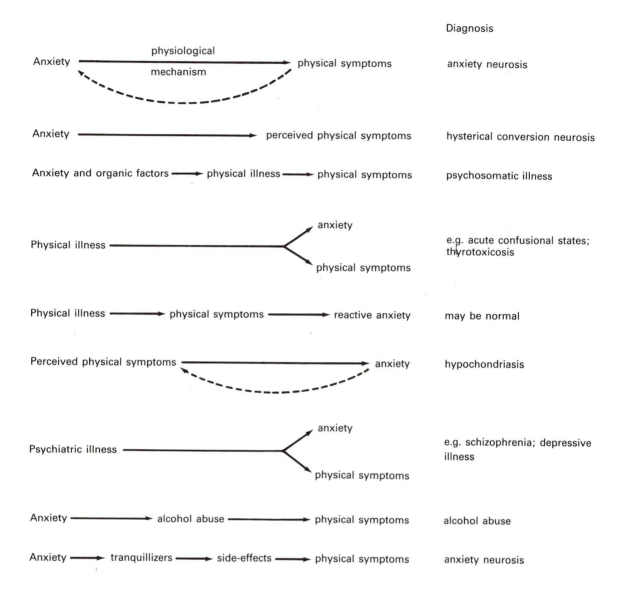

Figure 4 Relationship between anxiety and physical symptoms

PRIMARY ORGANIC PATHOLOGY

Organic illness may lead to psychological change in the following ways. Firstly, the patient may react to the illness, its symptoms or treatment with an alteration of mood, usually anxiety or depression, or both. This may influence the perception of the original physical symptoms, compliance with treatment and resolution of the disease process.

Secondly, the disease process may involve the brain, producing organic brain syndromes such as acute confusional states, dementia or functional (or symptomatic) psychoses. The latter often present with a change in mood which may be accompanied by paranoid ideation; they occur for example in endocrine and autoimmune disorders. In addition disturbance of the brain structure may lead to the development of epilepsy, which itself may present with psychological problems (see Chapter 20). Finally, the brain may be affected not only by structural or systemic disease but also by treatment, as with antihypertensive-induced depression and steroid psychoses.

PRIMARY PSYCHIATRIC ILLNESS

Physical symptoms secondary to psychiatric disorder can be classified into four groups.

1 Physical symptoms as a pathophysiological component of the emotional state
2 Physical symptoms, psychopathological in nature:
  a delusional
  b neurotic
3 Physical symptoms due to neglect or self-abuse
4 Physical symptoms as side-effects of psychiatric treatment

Pathophysiological component

Anxiety

People with anxiety states may present with somatic symptoms due to autonomic nervous system arousal. This is covered more fully in Chapter 13. The diagnosis is made by the nature of the symptoms and the presence of associated psychic symptoms of anxiety: the ability to reproduce the symptoms on voluntary overbreathing; their relief with reassurance; relaxation or sedative medication; and in some cases the presence of an anxiety-producing stress.

Depression

Depressive illnesses have a physical component possibly related to altered brain neurochemistry. Symptoms include early morning waking, significant alteration of appetite and weight, loss of libido, lethargy, constipation and psychomotor agitation and retardation. The diagnosis is made by the presence of other symptoms of depression (see Chapter 14).

Other disorders

Schizophrenia may be associated with movement disorders (see Chapter 3) and mania with overactivity.

Physical symptoms, psychopathological in nature

Delusional

Delusional ideas concerning bodily ill-health may be found in functional psychoses, and organic brain disease or in certain sensitive personalities. These include delusions of bodily change, as with the lady who said she was changing into a horse, as found in schizophrenia; and delusions or over-valued ideas of bodily ill-health sometimes seen in depressive illnesses. In these cases the patient is convinced that he is seriously ill and that the doctors are withholding the truth from him.

Nihilistic delusions include delusions in which the patient is convinced either that he is dead or that his insides are dead, rotting or absent. This is called Cotard's syndrome, and though classically found in depressive illnesses it may also occur in schizophrenia and organic psychoses.

Delusions of pregnancy may occur even where intercourse has not taken place, and are found in schizophrenia or affective psychosis. Patients may present with recurrent illnesses in which the delusion of pregnancy recurs. In all cases the diagnosis depends on the history and mental state, not just on the presenting symptoms.

Monosymptomatic delusional states — Dysmorphophobia

Some patients suffer from the isolated false belief, which may be delusional in extent, that there is something wrong with part of their body: for example, their nose is misshapen. The name dysmorphophobia has been given to the symptom, which usually results in an endless quest for medical opinions and corrective surgery, sometimes with disastrous results. It is found in sensitive personalities but may herald the onset of a schizophrenic illness (see Chapter 2). Dysmorphophobia is classified in DSM–III under Atypical Somatoform Disorder.

Neurotic

Most of the relevant disorders in this group are classified among the neuroses in ICD–9 but as a distinct category, the somatoform disorders, in DSM-III (see Table 21.1). As mentioned above, terminology in this area is confused, reflecting a lack of understanding of the basic concepts underlying the diagnoses used. The aetiological basis is usually a change in mood: anxiety, depression or both in response to a stressful precipitant; but the mechanism of production of physical symptoms differs according to the categories used. Figure 4 represents a simple scheme for the different links between anxiety and physical symptoms in different diagnostic categories. To further clarify this area, DSM–III operational guidelines are presented where appropriate.

Hypochondriasis

Hypochondriasis refers to excessive concern with health, either in general or with specific reference to one part of the body or mind. It may represent an exaggeration of the normal: for example every spot, however small and innocent, may represent a cancerous growth. This leads to frequent visits to the general practitioner with the resulting label

Table 21.1 Classification of physical symptoms due to neurotic psychopathology

ICD–9	DSM–III
Hypochondriasis (300.7)	Hypochondriasis (300.70) (Hypochondriacal neurosis)
Hysteria (300.1)	Conversion disorder (300.11) (Hysterical neurosis, conversion type)
Psychalgia (307.8)	Psychogenic pain disorder (307.80)
Other neurotic disorders (300.8) (including Briquet's disorder)	Somatization disorder (300.81)
	Atypical somatoform disorder (300.70(71)) (e.g. dysmorphophobia)

These disorders are known collectively in DSM–III as somatoform disorders.

of hypochondriasis. In addition symptoms may be retained long after organic pathology has healed, as in cardiac neurosis after myocardial infarction. It usually exists secondary to neurotic anxiety or depression, or as part of a personality disorder, though it may also occur in relation to one of the functional psychoses and, rarely, as an entity on its own.

In the DSM–III the diagnostic criteria for hypochondriasis include:

1 The predominant disturbance is an unrealistic interpretation of physical signs or sensations as abnormal, leading to preoccupation with the fear or belief of having serious disease

2 There is no evidence for the diagnosis of physical disorder to account for the above

3 The fear persists despite medical reassurance, and leads to impairment in work or social functions

4 It is not due to any other mental disorder, for example schizophrentia, affective disorder or somatization disorder

Hysteria

There has been much controversy surrounding the aetiology or indeed usefulness of the term hysteria which may be used in the following ways.

a To denote a person with theatrical, manipulative behaviour and difficulties in making relationships — hysterical personality disorder.

b As a lay term for highly emotional behaviour

c As a pejorative term — 'You're just being hysterical'

d To denote an exaggeration of physical symptoms for emotional reasons — hysterical overlay

e To denote the presence of physical or psychological symptoms as a response to stress but not due to pathophysiological processes — conversion hysteria, hysterical dissociative state

There are two different explanations for this disorder. The first is based on analytical principles and sees the disorder as being due to the conversion of anxiety to a physical or psychological symptom with a splitting off of part of the mental state — dissociation (see Hysterical Dissociative States, Chapter 19). The alternative hypothesis is based on social and behavioural factors and is associated with the development of sick-role behaviour. This suggests that at times of crisis people will develop symptoms, because this both avoids the stress and gets attention so that it becomes more advantageous to be ill than to be well.

According to both hypotheses, gain is important whether primary — as a way of dealing with distress by means of withdrawal; or secondary — as a way of getting extra attention.

The diagnosis should be made on positive grounds, and not just on the absence of a physical explanation for the symptoms, in order to avoid missing a true organic illness which may become apparent at a later date. Where doubts remain as to whether or not the symptoms are due to psychological disturbance, a working hypothesis should be set up and the patient treated accordingly. The past medical history is highly relevant and a life chart comparing physical symptoms with life events and psychological stresses is a useful diagnostic aid; as is a behavioural analysis of the symptoms, which can be achieved by asking the patient to keep a detailed diary.

In the DSM-III the diagnostic criteria of conversion disorder (hysterical neurosis, conversion type) are:

1 The predominant disturbance is a loss of or alteration in physical functioning suggesting a physical disorder
2 Psychological factors are involved in causing the symptoms as shown by one of the following:
   a a relationship in time to stress
   b the presence of primary gain
   c the presence of secondary gain
3 The symptom is not under voluntary control
4 It is not explicable on physical or pathophysiological grounds
5 The symptom is not limited to pain or sexual dysfunction
6 It is not due to somatization disorder or schizophrenia

Though patients with psychological illnesses may present with any physical symptoms pain is a particularly common one in such entities as atypical facial pain. In both ICD–9 and DSM–III this is classified separately from hysterical conversion neurosis: as psychalgia in ICD–9 and psychogenic pain disorder in DSM–III. In the latter the diagnostic criteria are largely similar to those of conversion disorder (see above).

Briquet's syndrome

In the DSM-III this is known as somatization disorder with the diagnostic criteria being:

a a history of physical symptoms of several years' duration beginning before the age of thirty
b complaints of fourteen or more symptoms for women (twelve for men) from a list of thirty-seven. The symptom must have led to taking medication (other than aspirin), alteration of life style or a consultation with a physician, and must not be adequately explained by physical disorder

Depressive equivalents

Some depressed patients present with physical symptoms for which there is no organic cause. Where they admit to being depressed the diagnosis presents little difficulty. However, some patients deny being depressed and the correct diagnosis is made by inference from associated symptoms such as early morning waking, loss of appetite, weight and libido, and is confirmed by the resolution of both the psychological and physical symptoms with the treatment of the depression.

Grief reaction

It is not uncommon for physical symptoms to occur in the bereaved. Though research has shown that true physical illness occurs more commonly after a bereavement, in some cases there is no organic basis for these physical symptoms. Often the bereaved may take on the symptoms of the illness from which the deceased died.

Cultural presentation

In the third world it is common for people with psychological problems to present with physical symptoms. This may be because the latter are more acceptable; a phenomenon found in other situations where there is a stigma, as with sexual disorders.

Post-traumatic neurosis

In some patients who have suffered an injury, symptoms may continue for many years without any organic pathology. They are often associated with a change in mood and personality, with anxiety and depression, irritability, loss of confidence and self-esteem and loss of libido; and also with physical symptoms such as headaches and dizziness. This probably represents a neurotic reaction to the stress of the accident, usually in a vulnerable personality, though malingering for compensation gain is a differential diagnosis.

Malingering

This is in fact extremely rare and as with any other diagnosis should only be made on positive grounds. In practice this either means catching the patient out or an admission on his behalf that he is not telling the truth.

Munchausen's syndrome

These patients travel from hospital to hospital presenting with graphic accounts of symptoms of severe organic illness, usually in the abdominal, respiratory or neurological system. The staff may be so taken in as to operate on these patients and often the diagnosis is only made by chance, for instance when a nurse or doctor on the ward recognises the patient from a previous hospital (see Chapter 17).

Physical symptoms due to neglect or self-abuse

Neglect

This may involve failure to take normal steps for nutrition, hydration and warmth, as in patients with dementia and chronic schizophrenia. Some patients with psychiatric illness may show poor compliance with treatment of any associated physical illnesses. Manic patients may be too busy with other activities to eat and may also suffer

from exhaustion; alcoholics may take in all their calories as alcohol with resulting vitamin B deficiency disorders; anorexics reduce their intake as part of their illness; patients with severe depression may fail to eat or drink; while those with paranoid illnesses may harbour paranoid delusious regarding food and drink.

Self-abuse

This includes deliberate self-harm as in the taking of overdoses and wrist-slashing, where the motive is usually not attempted suicide; as opposed to the severe injuries sustained in the failed suicide bid of a depressive, as a response to the voices of schizophrenia or as part of a drug-induced toxic state during which the patient is out of touch with reality. Both drug and alcohol abuse may lead to physical illness as may overeating and smoking. Anorexics may abuse laxatives or indulge in self-induced vomiting, both of which may lead to profound electrolyte imbalance. They may also, paradoxically, suffer as a result of too high a food intake at the beginning of treatment, which may cause ruptured stomachs. Patients with obsessive compulsive neuroses may indulge in extreme amounts of hand-washing with powerful antiseptic soap, resulting in skin disorders. Other patients may pick their skin or pull their hair out.

Physical illness following psychotropic drugs

Most of the psychotropic drugs in current use have side-effects which may be severe enough to cause the patient to present to his doctor. This is classically the case with the extrapyramidal side-effects of major tranquillizers: dystonia, parkinsonism, akathisea and tardive dyskinesea (see Chapter 3). Antidepressants of the tricyclic group usually have anticholinergic side-effects — for example dry mouth — which are not dangerous although they may be particularly troublesome to the patient; however, potentially lethal cardiac arrhythmias may also occur with these drugs. Monoamine oxidase inhibitors may lead to severe headaches due to potentially fatally raised blood pressure if the patient eats tyramine-containing foodstuffs, for example cheese, or concurrently takes other amine-containing drugs. Lithium may also cause both harmless and toxic symptoms, and propranolol may lead to heart failure or sudden death in asthmatics. Finally certain drugs may lead to withdrawal symptoms on discontinuation.

PSYCHOSOMATIC ILLNESS

It has long been known that many physical illnesses can be precipitated by stress. In the early days of psychosomatic medicine conflicting theories suggested that psychosomatic illness was either linked with specific personalities or caused by underlying neurotic conflicts. More recent research has suggested that both life events and personality traits are important psychological factors in the genesis and natural history of physical illness, but that rather than being sole aetiological agents they act in unison with organic factors. Thus stress is one of the risk factors in the development of ischaemic heart disease; others include smoking, hypertension, hypercholesterolaemia, diabetes and a family history of coronary artery disease.

Another example of the interplay between psychological and organic factors can be seen in asthma, one of the historical psychosomatic disorders. It is known that in seventy per cent of asthmatics psychological factors are important; the less obvious infection and allergy are, the more apparent is emotional distress. Discussion of emotionally disturbing material can produce an exacerbation in patients prone to developing asthma, and treatment must involve consideration of the psychological as well as the physical state of the patient. In other cases emotion leads to a disorder of function rather than pathological changes, e.g. irritable bowel disease.

Psychosomatic disorders, a fuller discussion of which is outside the remit of this book, are classified in ICD–9 under the heading 'Psychic Factors Associated with Disease Classified Elsewhere' 316. This is defined as 'Mental disturbances or psychic factors of any type thought to have played a major part in aetiology of physical conditions, usually involving tissue damage, classified elsewhere. The mental disturbance is usually mild and non-specific and psychic factors (worry, fear, conflict, etc) may be present without any overt psychiatric

disorder'. In DSM–III psychosomatic disorders are classified under the heading 'Psychological factors affecting physical conditions' 316.00. The diagnostic criteria for this diagnosis are:

a psychologically meaningful environmental stimuli are temporarily related to the initiation or exacerbation of a physical condition;

b the physical condition has either demonstrable organic pathology (e.g. rheumatoid arthritis) or a known pathophysiological process (migraine, headache, vomiting);

c the condition is not due to a somatoform disorder.

The assessment of the role of psychological factors in the development of physical illness necessitates a full and detailed psychiatric and medical history from both the patient and other informants, physical examination and appropriate investigations. Hospital or general practice medical notes give vital information about the previous medical history, and life charts and behavioural analyses are helpful diagnostic aids.

CASE HISTORY

ZOE THOMAS

Mrs Zoe Thomas was a 45-year-old bank clerk who was referred from the neurological department of a general hospital with a six-month history of difficulty in walking. Physical examination was normal as were all relevant investigations. Reassurance that there was no physical illness had been met with hostility as had the original suggestion of a psychiatric referral. However, her symptoms had led to increasing periods of absence from work and she was in danger of losing her job. Under great pressure she had finally agreed to see a psychiatrist.

During the interview Mrs Thomas strenuously denied any stresses. She enjoyed her job which she had had for ten years; this marriage, her second one, was perfect as had been her first one which had ended with the death of her husband a few months after developing cancer. She had two children from her first marriage, both of whom had married within the last three years. Her husband worked as a printer, his job was secure and there were no financial problems. She slept well and there had been no change in her appetite and no other symptoms of depression or anxiety.

She was an only child and had had a strict upbringing. Her father, a rather rigid bank manager, had never shown any affection towards her or her mother except at times of illness. Any show of feeling or of inability to cope was unacceptable. She had enjoyed school where she had made friends, but she had had difficulties with her gym teacher and recounted an episode where she developed pain in her legs which had led to her being excused from that particular class. The school doctor had found no cause for this pain which was only present on days when gym was held and had remitted completely at the end of that school year.

She had never seen a psychiatrist before nor had she needed psychotropic medication. Her only previous admission to hospital was soon after the death of her first husband, when she had been investigated for loss of balance. No organic cause had been found for this symptom which resolved over the following six to twelve months. When discussing her reaction to her bereavement she said that she had had to be the strong one for the sake of the children, but in any case she had always found it difficult to show her feelings.

Her husband was seen on his own and he confirmed that his wife had never worn her heart on her sleeve and had always coped well. However he had noticed that when things really got on top of her she sometimes went to bed for a day or two, suffering with aches and pains in her limbs, at which time the family rallied round and helped in the house. Like his wife, he denied any stresses at the present time. When the couple were seen together it was obvious that there was a great deal of tension in their relationship. This was because her husband, whom she had married three years previously, had been promoted at work. As a result of this he had had to work long hours and was frequently telephoned at home. In addition his wife was expected to do a great deal of entertaining and she was very resentful about this. Since she had become ill, she was no longer able to entertain and her husband had had to do the shopping, help with the housework and generally look after her.

Questions

What is the diagnosis and why?
Why has she reacted to stress in this way?
How would treatment confirm or refute the diagnosis?

The most likely diagnosis is a hysterical conversion neurosis. The evidence for this lies in the following points. Firstly, the absence of any abnormality on physical examination and investigations makes an organic cause of her symptoms extremely unlikely. Secondly there is the past history of response to stress with physical symptoms during her schooling, after her first husband's death at a time when she was unable to grieve openly, and to a lesser extent at other times during her life. Despite the denial of any stress by both her and her husband when seen independently, the joint interview revealed major marital problems. The fact that she functions by denial lends further support to a diagnosis of reaction to stress by the production of physical symptoms. There is evidence of both primary gain: her inability to entertain for her husband; and secondary gain: the increased attention that her husband had been paying her since she had been ill. The only other possible diagnoses are a depressive neurosis with the physical symptoms acting as a depressive equivalent, or an anxiety neurosis — the difficulty in walking may be due to anxiety or malingering. There are no associated symptoms of mood disturbance, and no positive evidence of malingering in the history.

During her childhood, feelings were not encouraged and attention was only given by her father to physical symptoms. In addition in one of her first confrontations with stress, namely doing gym at school, she had developed physical symptoms which had successfully allowed her to avoid this anxiety. Thus she might have learnt that physical symptoms were an acceptable, indeed the only acceptable, way of responding to stress and that they led to both primary and secondary gain. This pattern had been reinforced at other times in her life. Her current symptoms might thus be seen as the only way she can cope with the feelings of anxiety and anger engendered by the intrusiveness of her husband's work while at the same time they direct her husband's attention away from work towards her, thus encouraging her development of the sick role.

The diagnosis could be supported by showing that reduction of Mrs Thomas's symptoms follows the successful reorganization of her marriage, the ventilation of her angry feelings towards her husband, or both. At times when one remains uncertain after taking a detailed history whether physical symptoms are psychological in nature, the setting up of a hypothesis to explain the symptoms in psychological terms is often the only avenue open towards establishing a rational treatment plan. However it must be borne in mind that failure of resolution of symptoms with treatment does not necessarily refute the hypothesis, as it may be that no treatment, however correctly based theoretically, will be practically effective. Nevertheless at this stage it is important to re-evaluate the original hypothesis on which treatment was based. This may require further physical examination and investigation, or interviewing further informants or different combinations of informants. As shown in this history two people may give a very different story when seen independently from that which they give when they are seen together.

Appendix I: ICD–9★ classification of mental disorders

ICD–9 Classification of Mental Disorders (without inclusion and exclusion terms) from *Manual of the International Statistical Classification of Diseases, Injuries and Causes of Death*, Volume 1, World Health Organisation, Geneva, 1977.

Those categories in brackets are not included in DSM–III.

PSYCHOSES (290–299)

Organic psychotic conditions (290–294)

Senile and pre-senile organic psychotic conditions

290.0 Senile dementia, simple type
290.1 Pre-senile dementia
290.2 Senile dementia, depressed or paranoid type
290.3 Senile dementia with acute confusional state
290.4 Arteriosclerotic dementia
290.8 Other
290.9 Unspecified

Alcoholic psychoses

291.0 Delirium tremens
291.1 Korsakov's psychosis, alcoholic
291.2 Other alcoholic dementia
291.3 Other alcoholic hallucinosis
291.4 Pathological drunkenness
291.5 Alcoholic jealousy
291.8 Other
291.9 Unspecified

Drug psychoses

292.0 Drug withdrawal syndrome

ICD-10 is under preparation at the time of writing

292.1 Paranoid and/or hallucinatory states induced by drugs
292.2 [Pathological drug intoxication]
292.8 Other
292.9 Unspecified

Transient organic psychotic conditions

293.0 Acute confusional state
293.1 [Subacute confusional state]
293.8 Other
293.9 Unspecified

Other organic psychotic conditions (chronic)

294.0 Korsakov's psychosis (non-alcoholic)
294.1 Dementia in conditions classified elsewhere
294.8 Other
294.9 Unspecified

Other psychoses (295–299)

Schizophrenic psychoses

295.0 [Simple type]
295.1 Hebephrenic type
295.2 Catatonic type
295.3 Paranoid type
295.4 Acute schizophrenic episode
295.5 [Latent schizophrenia]
295.6 Residual schizophrenia
295.7 Schizoaffective type
295.8 Other
295.9 Unspecified

Affective psychoses

296.0 [Manic-depressive psychosis, manic type]

296.1 [Manic-depressive psychosis, depressed type]

296.2 Manic-depressive psychosis, circular type but currently manic

296.3 Manic-depressive psychosis, circular type but currently depressed

296.4 Manic- depressive psychosis, circular type, mixed

296.5 Manic-depressive psychosis, circular type, current condition not specified

296.6 Manic-depressive psychosis, other and unspecified

296.8 Other

296.9 Unspecified

Paranoid states

297.0 [Paranoid state, simple]

297.1 Paranoia

297.2 [Paraphrenia]

297.3 Induced psychosis

297.8 Other

297.9 Unspecified

Other non-organic psychoses

298.0 [Depressive type]

298.1 [Excitative type]

298.2 [Reactive confusion]

298.3 Acute paranoid reaction

298.4 [Psychogenic paranoid psychosis]

298.8 Other and unspecified reactive psychosis

298.9 Unspecified psychosis

Psychoses with origin specific to childhood

299.0 Infantile autism

299.1 [Disintegrative psychosis]

299.8 Other

299.9 Unspecified

NEUROTIC DISORDERS, PERSONALITY DISORDERS AND OTHER NON-PSYCHOTIC MENTAL DISORDERS (300–316)

Neurotic disorders

300.0 Anxiety states

300.1 Hysteria

300.2 Phobic state

300.3 Obsesive-compulsive disorder

300.4 Neurotic depression

300.5 [Neurasthenia]

300.6 Depersonalization syndrome

300.7 Hypochondriasis

300.8 Other

300.9 Unspecified

Personality disorders

301.0 Paranoid

301.1 Affective

301.2 Schizoid

301.3 [Explosive]

301.4 Anankastic

301.5 Hysterical

301.6 Asthenic

301.7 With predominantly sociopathic or asocial manifestations

301.8 Other

301.9 Unspecified

Sexual deviations and disorders

302.0 Homosexuality

302.1 Bestiality

302.2 Paedophilia

302.3 Transvestism

302.4 Exhibitionism

302.5 Transsexualism

302.6 Disorders of psychosexual indentity

302.7 Frigidity and impotence

302.8 Other

302.9 Unspecified

303   *Alcohol dependence syndrome.*

Drug dependence

304.0 Morphine type

304.1 Barbiturate type

304.2 [Cocaine]

304.3 Cannabis

304.4 Amphetamine type and other psycho-stimulants

304.5 [Hallucinogens]

304.6 Other

304.7 Combinations of morphine-type drug with any other

304.8   Combinations excluding morphine-type drug
304.9   Unspecified

Non-dependent abuse of drugs

305.0   Alcohol
305.1   Tobacco
305.2   Cannabis
305.3   Hallucinogens
305.4   Barbiturates and tranquillizers
305.5   Morphine type
305.6   Cocaine type
305.7   Amphetamine type
305.8   [Antidepressants]
305.9   Other, mixed, or unspecified

Physical conditions arising from mental factors

306.0   [Musculoskeletal]
306.1   [Respiratory]
306.2   [Cardiovascular]
306.3   [Skin]
306.4   [Gastrointestinal]
306.5   [Genitourinary]
306.6   [Endocrine]
306.7   [Organs of special sense]
306.8   [Other]
306.9   [Unspecified]

Special symptoms or syndromes not elsewhere classified

307.0   Stammering and stuttering
307.1   Anorexia nervosa
307.2   Tics
307.3   Stereotyped repetitive movements
307.4   Specific disorders of sleep
307.5   Other disorders of eating
307.6   Enuresis
307.7   Encopresis
307.8   Psychalgia
307.9   Other and unspecified

Acute reaction to stress

308.0   Predominant disturbance of emotions
308.1   Predominant disturbance of consciousness
308.2   Predominant psychomotor disturbance

308.3   Other
308.4   Mixed
308.9   Unspecified

Adjustment reaction

309.0   Brief depressive reaction
309.1   [Prolonged depressive reaction]
309.2   With predominant disturbance of other emotions
309.3   With predominant disturbance of conduct
309.4   With mixed disturbance of emotions and conduct
309.8   Other
309.9   Unspecified

Specific non-psychotic mental disorders following organic brain damage

310.0   [Frontal lobe syndrome]
310.1   Cognitive or personality change of other type
310.2   [Post-concussional syndrome]
310.8   Other
310.9   Unspecified

311   *[Depressive disorder, not elsewhere classified]*

Disturbance of conduct not elsewhere classified

312.0   Unsocialized disturbance of conduct
312.1   Socialized disturbance of conduct
312.2   Compulsive conduct disorder
312.3   [Mixed disturbance of conduct and emotions]
312.8   Other
312.9   Unspecified

Disturbance of emotions specific to childhood and adolescence

313.0   With anxiety and fearfulness
313.1   [With misery and unhappiness]
313.2   With sensitivity, shyness and social withdrawal
313.3   [Relationship problems]
313.8   Other or mixed
313.9   Unspecified

Hyperkinetic syndrome of childhood

314.0 Simple disturbance of activity and attention
314.1 [Hyperkinesis with developmental delay]
314.2 [Hyperkinetic conduct disorder]
314.8 Other
314.9 Unspecified

Specific delays in development

315.0 Specific reading retardation
315.1 Specific arithmetical retardation
315.2 Other specific learning difficulties
315.3 Developmental speech or language disorder
315.4 [Specific motor retardation]
315.5 Mixed developmental disorder

315.8 Other
315.9 Unspecified

316. *Psychic factors associated with diseases classified elsewhere*

MENTAL RETARDATION (317–319)

317. *Mild mental retardation*

Other specified mental retardation

318.0 Moderate mental retardation
318.1 Severe mental retardation
318.2 Profound mental retardation

319. *Unspecified mental retardation*

Appendix II: DSM III Classification: Axes I and II Categories and Codes

All official DSM-III codes and terms are included in ICD-9-CM. However, in order to differentiate those DSM-III categories that use the same ICD–9–CM codes, unoffical non-ICD–9 codes are provided in parentheses for use when greater specificity is necessary.

The long dashes indicate the need for a fifth-digit subtype or other qualifying term.

DISORDERS USUALLY FIRST EVIDENT IN INFANCY, CHILDHOOD OR ADOLESCENCE

Mental retardation

(Code in fifth digit: 1 = with other behavioural symptoms (requiring attention or treatment and that are not part of another disorder), 0 = without other behavioural symptoms)

317.0(x)	Mild mental retardation, _____
318.0(x)	Moderate mental retardation, _____
318.1(x)	Severe mental retardation, _____
318.2(x)	Profound mental retardation, _____
319.0(x)	Unspecified mental retardation, _____

Attention deficit disorder

314.01	with hyperactivity
314.00	without hyperactivity
314.80	residual type

Conduct disorder

312.00	undersocialized, aggressive
312.10	undersocialized, nonaggressive
312.23	socialized, aggressive
312.21	socialized, nonaggressive

312.90	atypical

Anxiety disorders of childhood or adolescence

309.21	Separation anxiety disorder
313.21	Avoidant disorder of childhood or adolescence
313.00	Overanxious disorder

Other disorders of infancy, childhood or adolescence

313.89	Reactive attachment disorder of infancy
313.22	Schizoid disorder of childhood or adolescence
313.23	Elective mutism
313.81	Oppositional disorder
313.82	Identity disorder

Eating disorders

307.10	Anorexia nervosa
307.51	Bulimia
307.52	Pica
307.53	Rumination disorder of infancy
307.50	Atypical eating disorder

Stereotyped movement disorders

307.21	Transient tic disorder
307.22	Chronic motor tic disorder
307.23	Tourette's disorder
307.20	Atypical tic disorder
307.30	Atypical stereotyped movement disorder

Other disorders with physical manifestations

307.00	Stuttering

307.60   Functional encopresis
307.70   Functional enuresis
307.46   Sleepwalking disorder
307.46   Sleep terror disorder (307.49)

Pervasive developmental disorders

(Code in fifth digit: 0 = full syndrome present, 1 = residual state)
299.0(x)   Infantile autism, _____
299.9(x)   Childhood onset pervasive developmental disorder, _____
299.8(x)   Atypical, _____

Specific developmental disorders   NOTE: these are coded on Axis II

315.00   Developmental reading disorder
315.10   Developmental arithmetic disorder
315.31   Developmental language disorder
315.39   Developmental articulation disorder
315.50   Mixed specific developmental disorder
315.90   Atypical specific developmental disorder

ORGANIC MENTAL DISORDERS

Section 1

Organic mental disorders whose aetiology or patho-physiological process is listed below (taken from the mental disorders section of ICD–9–CM).

Dementias arising in the senium and presenium

Primary degenerative dementia, senile onset,
290.30   with delirium
290.20   with delusions
290.21   with depression
209.00   uncomplicated
(Code in fifth digit: 1 = with delirium, 2 = with delusions, 3 = with depression, 0 = uncomplicated)
290.1(x)   Primary degenerative dementia, pre-senile, onset, _____
290.4(x)   Multi-infarct dementia, _____

Substance induced

Alcohol
303.00   intoxication

291.40   idiosyncratic intoxication
291.80   withdrawal
291.00   withdrawal delirium
291.30   hallucinosis
291.10   amnestic disorder
Code severity of dementia in fifth digit: 1 = mild, 2 = moderate, 3 = severe, 0 = unspecified)
291.2(x)   Dementia associated with alcoholism
Barbiturate or similarly acting sedative or hypnotic
305.40   intoxication (327.00)
292.00   withdrawal (327.01)
292.00   withdrawal delirium (327.02)
292.83   amnestic disorder (327.04)
Opioid
305.50   intoxication (327.10)
292.00   withdrawal (327.11)
Cocaine
305.60   intoxication (327.20)
Amphetamine or similarly acting sympathomimetic
305.70   intoxication (327.30)
292.81   delirium (327.32)
292.11   delusional disorder (327.35)
292.00   withdrawal (327.31)
Phencyclidine (PCP) or similarly acting arylcyclohexylamine
305.90   intoxication (327.40)
292.81   delirium (327.42)
292.90   mixed organic mental disorder (327.49)
Hallucinogens
305.30   hallucinosis (327.56)
292.11   delusional disorder (327.55)
292.84   affective disorder (327.57)
Cannabis
305.20   intoxication (327.60)
292.11   delusional disorder (327.65)
Tobacco
292.00   withdrawal (327.71)
Caffeine
305.90   intoxication (327.80)
Other or unspecified substance
305.90   intoxication (327.90)
292.00   withdrawal (327.91)
292.81   delirium (327.92)
292.82   dementia (327.93)
292.83   amnestic disorder (327.94)
292.11   delusional disorder (327.95)
292.12   hallucinosis (327.96)
292.84   affective disorder (327.97)

292.89   personality disorder (327.98)
292.90   atypical or mixed organic mental disorder (327.99)

Section 2

Organic brain syndromes whose aetiology or pathophysiology process is either noted as an additional diagnosis from outside the mental disorders section of ICD-9-CM or is unknown.

293.00   Delirium
294.10   Dementia
294.00   Amnestic syndrome
293.81   Organic delusional syndrome
293.82   Organic hallucinosis
293.83   Organic affective syndrome
310.10   Organic personality syndrome
294.80   Atypical or mixed organic brain syndrome

SUBSTANCE USE DISORDERS

(Code in fifth digit: 1 = continuous, 2 = episodic, 3 = in remission, 0 = unspecified)

305.0(x)   Alcohol abuse, _____
303.9(x)   Alcohol dependence (Alcoholism), ____
305.4(x)   Barbiturate or similarly acting sedative or hypnotic abuse, _____
304.1(x)   Barbiturate or similarly acting sedative or hypnotic dependence, _____
305.5(x)   Opioid abuse, _____
304.0(x)   Opioid dependence, _____
305.6(x)   Cocaine abuse, _____
305.7(x)   Amphetamine or similarly acting sympathomimetic abuse, _____
304.4(x)   Amphetamine or similarly acting sympathomimetic dependence, _____
305.9(x)   Phencyclidine (PCP) or similarly acting arylcyclohexylamine abuse, _____ (328.4x)
305.3(x)   Hallucinogen abuse, _____
305.2(x)   Cannabis abuse, _____
304.3(x)   Cannabis dependence, _____
305.1(x)   Tobacco dependence, _____
305.9(x)   Other, mixed or unspecified substance abuse, _____
304.6(x)   Other specified substance dependence, _____
304.9(x)   Unspecified substance dependence, ____

304.7(x)   Dependence on combination of opioid and other nonalcoholic substance, ____
304.8(x)   Dependence on combination of substances, excluding opioids and alcohol, _____

SCHIZOPHRENIC DISORDERS

(Code in fifth digit: 1 = subchronic, 2 = chronic, 3 = subchronic with acute exacerbation, 4 = chronic with acute exacerbation, 5 = in remission, 0 = unspecified)
Schizophrenia
295.1(x)   disorganized, _____
295.2(x)   catatonic, _____
295.3(x)   paranoid, _____
295.9(x)   undifferentiated, _____
295.6(x)   residual, _____

PARANOID DISORDERS

297.10   Paranoia
297.30   Shared paranoid disorder
298.30   Acute paranoid disorder
297.90   Atypical paranoid disorder

PSYCHOTIC DISORDERS NOT ELSEWHERE CLASSIFIED

295.40   Schizophreniform disorder
298.80   Brief reactive psychosis
295.70   Schizoaffective disorder
298.90   Atypical psychosis

NEUROTIC DISORDERS

These are included in Affective, Anxiety, Somatoform, Dissociative and Psychosexual Disorders. In order to facilitate the identification of the categories that in DSM-II were grouped together in the class of Neuroses, the DSM-II terms are included separately in parentheses after the corresponding categories. These DSM-II terms are included in ICD-9-Cm and therefore are acceptable as alternatives to the recommended DSM-III terms that precede them.

AFFECTIVE DISORDERS

Major affective disorders

Code *major depressive* episode in fifth digit: 6 = in remission, 4 = with psychotic features (the unofficial non-ICD-9-CM fifth digit 7 may be used instead to indicate that the psychotic features are mood-incongruent), 3 = with melancholia, 2 = without melancholia, 0 = unspecified.

Code *manic* episode in fifth digit: 6 = in remission, 4 = with psychotic features (the unofficial non-ICD-9-CM fifth digit 7 may be used instead to indicate that the psychotic features are mood-incongruent), 2 = without psychotic features, 0 = unspecified.

Bipolar disorder
296.6(x)   mixed, _____
296.4(x)   manic, _____
296.5(x)   depressed, _____
Major depression
296.2(x)   single episode, _____
296.3(x)   recurrent, _____

Other specific affective disorders

301.13   Cyclothymic disorder
300.40   Dysthymic disorder (or Depressive neurosis)

Atypical affective disorders

296.70   Atypical bipolar disorder
296.82   Atypical depression

ANXIETY DISORDERS

Phobic disorders (or Phobic neuroses)
300.21   Agoraphobia with panic attacks
300.22   Agoraphobia without panic attacks
300.23   Social phobia
300.29   Simple phobia
Anxiety states (or Anxiety neuroses)
300.01   Panic disorder
300.02   Generalized anxiety disorder
300.30   Obsessive compulsive disorder (or Obsessive compulsive neurosis)
Post traumatic stress disorder
308.30   acute

309.81   chronic or delayed
300.00   Atypical anxiety disorder

SOMATOFORM DISORDERS

300.81   Somatization disorder
300.11   Coversion disorder (or Hysterical neurosis, conversion type)
307.80   Psychogenic pain disorder
300.70   Hypochondriasis (or Hypochondriacal neurosis)
300.70   Atypical somatoform disorder (300.71)

DISSOCIATIVE DISORDERS (OR HYSTERICAL NEUROSES, DISSOCIATIVE TYPE)

300.12   Psychogenic amnesia
300.13   Psychogenic fugue
300.14   Multiple personality
300.60   Depersonalization disorder (or Depersonalization neurosis)
300.15   Atypical dissociative disorder

PSYCHOSEXUAL DISORDERS

Gender identity disorders

(Indicate sexual history in the fifth digit of Transsexualism code: 1 = asexual, 2 = homosexual, 3 = heterosexual, 0 = unspecified)
302.5(x)   Transsexualism, _____
302.60   Gender identity disorder of childhood
302.85   Atypical gender identity disorder

Paraphilias

302.81   Fetishism
302.30   Transvestism
302.10   Zoophilia
302.20   Paedophilia
302.40   Exhibitionism
302.82   Voyeurism
302.83   Sexual masochism
302.84   Sexual sadism
302.90   Atypical paraphilia

Psychosexual dysfunctions

302.71   Inhibited sexual desire
302.72   Inhibited sexual excitement
302.73   Inhibited female orgasm
302.74   Inhibited male orgasm
302.75   Premature ejaculation
302.76   Functional dyspareunia
306.51   Functional vaginismus
302.70   Atypical psychosexual dysfunction

Other psychosexual disorders

302.00   Ego-dystonic homosexuality
302.89   Psychosexual disorder not elsewhere classified

FACTITIOUS DISORDERS

300.16   Factitious disorder with psychological symptoms
301.51   Chronic factitious disorder with physical symptoms
300.19   Atypical factitious disorder with physical symptoms

DISORDERS OF IMPULSE CONTROL NOT ELSEWHERE CLASSIFIED

312.31   Pathological gambling
312.32   Kleptomania
312.33   Pyromania
312.34   Intermittent explosive disorder
312.35   Isolated explosive disorder
312.39   Atypical impulsive control disorder

ADJUSTMENT DISORDER

309.00   with depressed mood
309.24   with anxious mood
309.28   with mixed emotional features
309.30   with disturbance of conduct
309.40   with mixed disturbance of emotions and conduct
309.23   with work (or academic) inhibition

309.83   with withdrawal
309.90   with atypical features

PSYCHOLOGICAL FACTORS AFFECTING PHYSICAL CONDITION

Specify physical condition on Axis III.
316.00   Psychological factors affecting physical condition

PERSONALITY DISORDERS

NOTE: These are coded on Axis II
301.00   Paranoid
301.20   Schizoid
301.22   Schizoptypal
301.50   Histrionic
301.81   Narcissistic
301.70   Antisocial
301.83   Borderline
301.82   Avoidant
301.60   Dependent
301.40   Compulsive
301.84   Passive-Aggressive
301.89   Atypical, mixed or other personality disorder

V CODES FOR CONDITIONS NOT ATTRIBUTABLE TO A MENTAL DISORDER THAT ARE A FOCUS OF ATTENTION OR TREATMENT

V65.20   Malingering
V62.89   Borderline intellectual functioning (V62.88)
V71.01   Adult antisocial behaviour
V71.02   Childhood or adolescent antisocial behaviour
V62.30   Academic problem
V62.20   Occupational problem
V62.82   Uncomplicated bereavement
V15.81   Noncompliance with medical treatment
V62.89   Phase of life problem or other life circumstance problem
V61.10   Marital problem

V61.20   Parent-child problem
V61.80   Other specified family circumstances
V62.81   Other interpersonal problem

ADDITIONAL CODES

300.90   Unspecified mental disorder (nonpsychotic)
V71.09   No diagnosis or condition on Axis I
799.90   Diagnosis or condition deferred on Axis
         I
V71.09   No diagnosis on Axis II
799.90   Diagnosis deferred on Axis II

Index